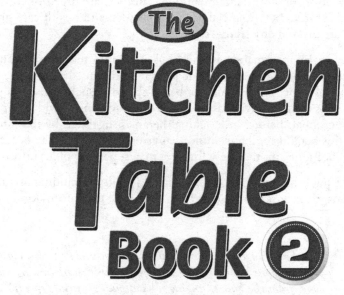

The Kitchen Table Book 2

All New Kitchen Cures and
Pantry Potions for Every
Health and Household Problem

Publisher's Note

This book is intended for general information only. It does not constitute medical, legal, or financial advice or practice. The editors of FC&A have taken careful measures to ensure the accuracy and usefulness of the information in this book. While every attempt has been made to assure accuracy, errors may occur. Some websites, addresses, and telephone numbers may have changed since printing. We cannot guarantee the safety or effectiveness of any advice or treatments mentioned. Readers are urged to consult with their professional financial advisors, lawyers, and health care professionals before making any changes.

Any health information in this book is for information only and is not intended to be a medical guide for self-treatment. It does not constitute medical advice and should not be construed as such or used in place of your doctor's medical advice. Readers are urged to consult with their health care professionals before undertaking therapies suggested by the information in this book, keeping in mind that errors in the text may occur as in all publications and that new findings may supersede older information.

The publisher and editors disclaim all liability (including any injuries, damages, or losses) resulting from the use of the information in this book.

Let the message of Christ dwell among you richly as you teach and admonish one another with all wisdom through psalms, hymns, and songs from the Spirit, singing to God with gratitude in your hearts.
Colossians 3:16 (NIV)

FC&A Medical Publishing®
103 Clover Green
Peachtree City, GA 30269

Produced by the staff of FC&A
ISBN 978-1-935574-64-4

Table of Contents

Allium vegetables

Pungent protection for your joints

You can smell an allium from a mile away. This family of vegetables, which includes onions, chives, garlic, scallions, shallots,
and leeks, is famous not only for its pungent flavors, but its
potent aromas.

And while these six foods might leave you with a mild case of
bad breath, if you're over age 55, you should be eating them
regularly. Adding alliums to your diet will help ward off some
of the most dreaded age-related diseases, like cancer, heart disease, and Alzheimer's.

To launch into the wonderful world of health-giving alliums,
find out how they will stop arthritis pain in its tracks.

Soothe your RA aches with quercetin. Inflamed, painful joints
caused by rheumatoid arthritis (RA) make even the simplest
everyday tasks unbearable. But there's a natural chemical in
onions, called quercetin, that acts as an anti-inflammatory to
stop this pain.

In a small study, researchers found 500 milligrams of quercetin
supplements daily helped relieve RA symptoms after only
eight weeks.

You'll get the most quercetin from red onions, which have a
mild flavor and are perfect for eating raw.

Sulfur compounds defend against OA. The nutrients in alliums do more than just soothe swelling and pain. They can actually keep you from developing the degenerative joint disease osteoarthritis (OA), in the first place. After examining the diets of twins, researchers from the public research university King's College London discovered those who ate the most allium vegetables were the least likely to get OA. Experts think the sulfur compounds, which give alliums their unique flavors, act as antioxidants to protect your cartilage.

Bone up on these surprising sources of vitamins. If you have low levels of vitamins C and K, you're gambling with your chances of developing OA, given the link between a deficiency in your diet and higher rates of knee arthritis.

- Onions probably don't come to mind when you think about vitamin C, but they contain a decent amount. Half a cup of raw, chopped onions gives you 10 percent of your recommended daily intake. Next time you have a salad or a sandwich, add a few onion slices.

- Alliums are also a tasty way to get your vitamin K. For instance, one leek contains more than half your daily dose. Better yet, reach for a scallion. Just one of these small spring onions has even more vitamin K than an entire leek. Make sure you eat the whole plant, though. You'll be wasting nutrients if you skip the dark green tops.

A royal cure for the disease of kings. Gout has long been known as the rich man's disease because it goes hand in hand with extravagant, meat-heavy diets. It dates all the way back to the ancient Egyptians, who first described this painful form of arthritis, and were, perhaps, on to a cure thousands of years before the rest of the world — archeologists have found onions buried with pharaohs and images of onions painted on the walls of pyramids. Now, researchers are beginning to discover the healing powers of these ancient vegetables.

Gout is caused by uric acid, which builds up and forms tiny crystals in your joints. Your body tries to protect you, a bit like how an oyster tries to protect itself from a loose grain of sand. Only instead of a pearl, you get swollen, inflamed joints.

A recent study showed quercetin can lower the amount of uric acid in your body. People in the study took quercetin supplements, but if you'd rather get it naturally, you'll need to eat about two-thirds of a red onion daily.

So to cool your burning joints, stock your pantry with onions and garlic — just pick up a few breath mints, too.

The all-natural way to keep garlic breath at bay

Brush your teeth a hundred times, but you'll never get rid of garlic breath by bedtime. That's because the source of the smell isn't coming from your mouth — it's coming from your lungs. The compounds that give garlic its powerful scent don't actually get digested. Instead, your body absorbs them and they are only released through your breath and sweat.

But don't worry, you can fight the funk. Apples contain an enzyme that neutralizes the odor-causing chemicals in garlic. So whenever you're eating a garlicky meal, add a few slices on the side. Heating destroys these enzymes though, so make sure you eat your apples raw.

Crush your risk of Alzheimer's with these powerful plants

Every garlic and onion lover has to make the impossible decision — eat a bland dinner or wind up banished to the far end of the sofa. But if you spread the news these aromatic plants can prevent Alzheimer's disease (AD), perhaps you'll convince the most ardent allium haters to chow down with you.

Aged garlic attacks AD-causing compounds. Whenever you get a cut or scrape, your body heals itself. And your brain is no different. If it's hurt by pollutants, trauma, or age-related stress, it activates microglial cells, your natural form of damage control. These cells gather and multiply to stop injuries from getting worse and to kick-start the healing process.

But there's a problem. Microglial cells also produce nitric oxide (NO), a chemical compound which, in excess, experts think leads to AD.

Researchers from the University of Missouri believe one secret to preventing this dangerous domino effect is in garlic — specifically aged garlic. A compound created during the aging process, called fructosyl arginine (FruArg), actually stops the production of NO. If you can't find aged garlic extract as a supplement at your local store, it's available for sale online.

A natural way to get this compound is from an exotic ingredient called black garlic. This sweet, mellow spice is just regular garlic that's been aged until the cloves turn black. Track it down at local grocers or buy black garlic on the internet.

Onions combat mind-dulling inflammation. When bacteria, viruses, or other irritants attack, your body reacts with inflammation, a natural way to start the healing process. But if inflammation becomes a chronic problem, it can lead to serious conditions like diabetes, cancer, and AD.

Researchers in the United Kingdom think the key to beating chronic inflammation could be in the produce section of your grocery store. Onions — as well as apples and green tea — contain natural chemicals called polyphenols that target and control chronic inflammation.

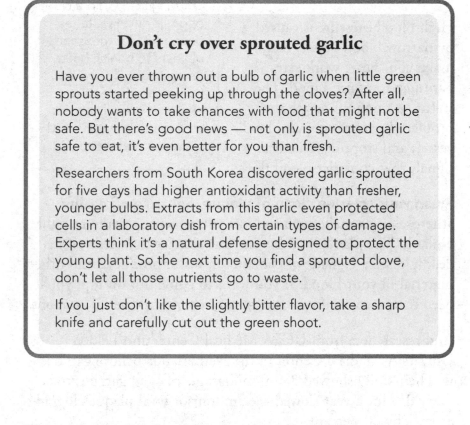

Don't cry over sprouted garlic

Have you ever thrown out a bulb of garlic when little green sprouts started peeking up through the cloves? After all, nobody wants to take chances with food that might not be safe. But there's good news — not only is sprouted garlic safe to eat, it's even better for you than fresh.

Researchers from South Korea discovered garlic sprouted for five days had higher antioxidant activity than fresher, younger bulbs. Extracts from this garlic even protected cells in a laboratory dish from certain types of damage. Experts think it's a natural defense designed to protect the young plant. So the next time you find a sprouted clove, don't let all those nutrients go to waste.

If you just don't like the slightly bitter flavor, take a sharp knife and carefully cut out the green shoot.

This savory herb safeguards your heart

Dozens of vitamins and supplements promise to heal your heart, but trying to keep up with them all can be overwhelming. If you're after something that can attack atherosclerosis, bring down your blood pressure, crush blood clots, and clobber cholesterol, look no further. Garlic is the one plant that can do it all.

Take the edge off of high blood pressure. You can keep your arteries open and flowing freely by just adding garlic to your daily menu. Its sulfur compounds are responsible for the pungent smell and sharp taste, but they also give garlic heart-healing powers.

High blood pressure is caused by narrow blood vessels that make your heart work extra hard just to pump blood. The sulfur compounds attack the problem by relaxing your blood vessels and stopping chemical signals that constrict blood flow.

If you feel a cold coming on, don't reach for the orange juice. Grab a clove of garlic, instead. It has been used for thousands of years to banish bacteria and fight viruses, and now researchers have proven it actually boosts your immune system and prevents infections.

Flush your arteries clean of plaque. Squaring off against atherosclerosis makes you feel like you're getting ready to fight Goliath. The plaque buildup in your arteries that defines this deadly disease is made of cholesterol, waste products, and other material in your blood. If you want to come out on top, you'll need to arm yourself with one of nature's most powerful weapons.

And researchers from UCLA Medical Center and Leiden University Medical Center in the Netherlands believe garlic is it. Their study showed 2,400 milligrams of aged garlic extract every day for a year slowed the amount of total plaque clogging arteries by 80 percent.

In addition, the sulfur compounds in garlic keep low-density lipoprotein (LDL) cholesterol from oxidizing. This chemical reaction is triggered by unhealthy habits — like a diet high in trans fats or smoking — and causes tissue damage and the buildup of plaque inside your arteries.

Your microwave holds the secret to tear-free onions

It's nearly impossible to escape the burning, stinging tears that make chopping onions such a nightmare. Tricks like chewing gum, lighting candles, and cutting onions under cold, running water just leave you crying and feeling silly. But there's one tool in your kitchen guaranteed to ward off the waterworks — your microwave.

The reason you cry when you're cutting onions is because they're actually trying to fight back. When onions are damaged, they release enzymes that produce eye-watering sulfur gases.

However, you can destroy those pesky enzymes by heating them up. So before you start slicing, trim off the ends of your onion and microwave it for 30 to 45 seconds on full power.

Blood clots beware — garlic is here. It's a bird, it's a plane, it's a … bulb of garlic? Garlic isn't the star of a blockbuster movie, but it is a nutritional superhero, especially since multiple studies show it could be the key to preventing deadly blood clots.

It all starts with cell fragments called platelets, which are a bit like natural Band-Aids. Whenever these little disks think you're injured, they change into spiny balls that clump together and form clots to stop the bleeding. When plaque damages your arteries, however, too many clots form. They further block your blood flow and sometimes break away to cause strokes and heart attacks. Fortunately, garlic can swoop in and save the day.

A recent study published in *The Journal of Nutrition* reports aged garlic extract stops blood from clotting by keeping the platelets from changing their shape and sticking together.

This might be a problem if you take blood thinners, like warfarin, however, so make sure you talk to your doctor before going all in on garlic.

Ramp up your cancer protection with alliums

The distinct flavors and smells of allium vegetables made them prized ingredients in ancient remedies. Some people used onions to treat everything from hair loss to the flu, and the ancient Egyptians believed garlic could cure 32 separate illnesses. Now researchers are finally beginning to peel back the layers and see the truth behind these myths. While these plants won't bring back your curly locks, they will offer potent protection against some of the most dangerous cancers.

- A look at over 20 studies confirmed the link — people who eat the most onions, scallions, leeks, and garlic are much less likely to develop stomach and colon cancers.

- Researchers studied more than 800 Chinese for two years, and discovered that eating raw garlic at least twice a week cut the risk of lung cancer in half, compared to those who ate no garlic.

Eating raw garlic isn't for everyone, but heating it immediately after chopping destroys a lot of the health benefits. Fortunately, there's a solution. Just crush your garlic five to 15 minutes before cooking. This gives allicin, one of the sulfur compounds responsible for garlic's miraculous powers, plenty of time to form.

The secret behind these amazing powers may be alliums' unique sulfur compounds. These chemicals, which give the plants their special taste, combat cancer on two fronts. First they protect your body from cancer-causing substances and ward off other irritants, then they seek out and attack existing cancerous cells.

A tasty way to jump-start your weight loss

Trendy diets always seem promising, but they just set you up to fail. If you've tried one before, you're probably suspicious of anything that claims it will make losing weight easy. Especially if it's as simple as eating a few onions. As silly as that sounds, it just might work. That's because it's not a weight-loss plan dreamed up by tabloids. Instead, it's based on a new study conducted by South Korean researchers.

Quercetin, a natural chemical found in onions, was the star of this particular investigation. Researchers divided people into two groups. One took a placebo pill every day, and the other a supplement containing 100 milligrams of quercetin — the amount in about a third of an onion.

After 12 weeks, researchers discovered those who took the supplement lost significantly more weight than the other group. And it gets even better. They also lost inches from their waist, hips, and thighs, as well as total body fat. It seems quercetin affects how your body breaks down and stores fat in your cells, a process called lipid metabolism.

So if you're looking to drop a few pounds, skip the crazy cleanses and pick up a few onions. Just make sure you don't waste the outer layers — they have more quercetin than the core.

Almonds

A natural way to end sleepless nights

Want to sleep sounder and wake up refreshed every day? Add almonds to your diet — the sleep aid you can take every night to help you face the world every morning.

You've probably heard of melatonin, the supplement many people take to relieve jet lag. But did you know melatonin is also a hormone your body makes? It's true.

Melatonin is secreted by the pineal gland located in the center of your brain. It directs your body's natural clock throughout your sleep-and-wake cycles, also called your circadian rhythm. But your body produces less melatonin as you get older, making it more difficult for you to enjoy a good night's rest. That's where almonds come in.

Melatonin occurs naturally in plant-based foods like almonds. In fact, research shows getting melatonin from food may help you doze off faster and snooze more soundly.

Melatonin does more than just help you sleep. It's great for reducing blood pressure, too. Your BP naturally rises during the day and falls at night. Eating melatonin-rich foods like almonds before bedtime can make your nighttime numbers drop even more. The result? A greater day-night blood pressure difference, which helps protect your heart.

Melatonin is in ample supply in other foods, too. Check out these drinks, snacks, and spices you can easily add to your diet.

- fenugreek
- flaxseeds
- goji (lycium) berries
- mustard seeds
- raspberries
- orange bell peppers
- tomatoes
- walnuts
- tart cherries or tart cherry juice

Good quality sleep not only makes you feel rested and full of energy, but when you get enough, it slows down aging, too. So grab an almond snack, and see you in the morning.

A handful of almonds = a heart full of almond joy

True or false — popping pills is the only way to get your high cholesterol and high blood pressure under control. If you answered true, you'd be wrong. Almonds, in fact, can slash both.

Keep your cholesterol in check. Multiple studies show the promising effects almonds have on cholesterol.

- People who snacked on eight almonds before breakfast every day for 12 weeks raised their HDL cholesterol. No worries, HDL is the good kind.

- Another study shows noshing on almonds every day works alongside statin therapy to lower bad cholesterol even more than taking the drug by itself. This could be helpful if you don't want to take a higher statin dose to reach your goal.

- What's more, researchers looked at the results of 27 studies and found that almonds also reduced bad LDL cholesterol and cut the risk of heart disease.

Banish high blood pressure. British researchers worked with a mix of healthy men and men with heart disease risk factors, like excess body weight or high blood pressure. One group ate their normal diet, while the other snacked on 40 almonds every day.

After a month, the almond eaters had higher amounts of antioxidants in their bloodstream, lower blood pressure, and better blood flow.

Researchers give credit for both these heart-healthy changes, lower cholesterol and blood pressure, to all the nutritious compounds in almonds — like fiber, vitamin E, minerals, good-for-you fats, and helpful plant sterols and flavonoids.

Added bonus — even though every almond has seven calories, many almond eaters in these controlled studies also lost weight. Experts say a trimmer you makes for a healthier heart.

Lose the jiggle around your middle

"Less is more," so they say, but when it comes to almonds, "more is less." The more almonds you munch on, the less food you eat and the less body fat you carry. That sounds like a good deal, but don't go nuts — a handful is all you need for a leaner, healthier you.

That's what researchers learned when they pitted two choles-terol-lowering diets against each other. Both contained the same amount of saturated fat, but one included a snack of 35 almonds and the other a banana muffin with similar calories. Everyone in the study was middle-aged, overweight, and had high cholesterol. At the end of 12 weeks, neither group had lost or gained weight, but only the almond eaters trimmed stubborn inches from those problem areas — their thighs and bellies.

Experts think it's all the fabulous nutrients in almonds, like fiber, protein, and healthy unsaturated fat, that make it a fat-trimming dynamo. These also tend to make you feel full, so you don't go looking for extra calories.

Dr. Michael Greger, a leading authority on health and nutrition, offers another theory. Yes, almonds curb your appetite, he says, and that's one reason why you eat less. But he also suggests people who eat almonds don't chew them well, so they end up flushing about one-third of their calories down the toilet. That could be another reason why people who eat almonds don't gain weight, says Greger.

Still, if you want to add almonds to your diet, take calories into consideration. One almond has about seven.

Almond milk — a nondairy delight

Almond milk isn't just the delicious drink *du jour* for hip vegans. It was popular back in the Middle Ages because it didn't spoil as quickly as dairy milk. Today, people reach for it as a healthy alternative to cow's milk. Here's why.

Although that wonderful liquid you've spent decades pouring over your cereal is brimming with great nutrients like bone-healthy calcium and vitamin D, plus proteins that support strong muscles, research shows cow's milk is also linked to prostate and aggressive ovarian cancer. In addition, you've probably heard most is loaded with hormones, which scientists fear could promote cancerous tumors. That's scary. Is it time to try something new?

So — should you sip it or skip it? Like all good things, almond milk has its downsides, too. Through processing it loses most of its protein, and the sweetened varieties have added sugar.

Plus, some contain a small amount of carrageenan, a seaweed compound also used in chocolate milk, ice cream, and salad dressings. This FDA-approved additive keeps a gritty layer of ground almonds from settling at the bottom of your glass and helps give almond milk its creaminess. Some say carrageenan can cause inflammation in your digestive tract, so check labels for this additive if you struggle with tummy woes.

How does one cup of your favorite milk measure up?

Type of milk	Calories	Total fat grams	Calcium % Daily Value
Unsweetened almond milk	30	2.5	45
Sweetened almond milk	60	2.5	45
Unsweetened vanilla almond milk	30	2.5	45
Sweetened vanilla almond milk	80-90	2.5	45
Whole dairy milk	146	7.9	28
2% dairy milk	122	4.8	29
1% dairy milk	102	2.4	29
Fat-free or skim dairy milk	86	0.4	30

Moo-ve over dairy, nut milk is here to stay. If you're lactose intolerant, almond milk makes a delicious substitute in cereals, smoothies, and coffee. It also promotes heart health, because it contains no bad fat or cholesterol. What's more, studies show almond milk may battle prostate cancer.

What about strong bones? After all, that's what regular milk is known for. No problem. Almond milk has plenty of added calcium and vitamin D. In fact, ounce for ounce, the nutty beverage gives you more calcium than moo juice.

As for price, you won't go broke. A refrigerated half-gallon of almond milk sells for almost the same as a half-gallon of regular milk.

Whip up a better butter

Does the thought of chewing almonds make your teeth hurt? Reach for almond butter, instead. It's chock-full of the same protein, fiber, vitamins, minerals, and healthy fats as the nuts, but without the crunch. Just check labels before you buy. Some brands have more added salt and sugar than others.

Better yet, make your own.

1. Place 4 cups of almonds in a food processor and blend until a paste forms.

2. Add 1/2 teaspoon salt or 1 teaspoon honey per cup of nuts, if desired, and pulse until blended.

3. Store in an airtight container in the fridge for up to two months.

For extra flavor, roast your almonds in a single layer on a baking sheet for eight to 10 minutes at 375 degrees before processing.

Add this delicious and healthy almond butter to your morning smoothie, stir it into puréed soups, or whisk into a basic vinaigrette. Get creative and enjoy.

Go a little nuts to battle brittle bones

About 54 million Americans suffer from osteoporosis or weakened bones that put them at risk of falls and fractures. That's the bad news. The good news is, you can do something about it simply by snacking on almonds.

Your skeleton constantly goes through a renewing process in which cells, called osteoclasts, break down and eat bone. No worries — like a construction crew, you also have cells that rebuild your bones. The builders are called osteoblasts.

Osteoporosis happens when these cells get out of whack, and you've got more bone eating than bone building going on. It's most common in menopausal women due to hormone changes.

Now that you understand how bones become brittle, you can better understand how almonds help.

A team of researchers decided to put almonds under the microscope. They exposed bone cells to blood samples taken four hours after a group of people ate test meals, one of which included about 50 almonds. Guess what happened? Blood from the almond-eaters stopped osteoclasts from forming and functioning.

The study doesn't explain why almonds keep osteoclasts in check, but here's what experts do know. Almonds are a rich source of two bone-healthy minerals, calcium and magnesium, with 1 ounce, about 23 almonds, delivering 75 milligrams of each. That's a good start on your recommended daily intake.

Enjoy beauty in a nutshell

Don't spend a pretty penny on lotions and potions. When it comes to radiant-looking skin, what you put *in* your body is just as important as what you put on it. Say hello to almonds and kiss aging skin good-bye.

Almonds are loaded with a form of vitamin E called a-tocopherol, a powerful antioxidant. It zaps skin-damaging free radicals and protects against skin cancer.

What's more, almonds are full of flavonoids, plant compounds that:

- scavenge free radicals.
- filter out damaging ultraviolet rays.
- act as anti-inflammatories.
- protect cells from harm and cell death.
- guard against skin cancer.
- block DNA damage.

Want more almonds? Nutcracking good ideas

Don't get stuck in a nut rut. Almonds are more versatile than you think.

- Boost the body and texture of vinaigrettes with finely chopped blanched almonds.
- Add slivered almonds to cooked grains like quinoa or stir-fried dishes.
- Use almond oil for any recipe that requires high heat like browning or searing.
- Coat baked fish or chicken with almond meal or flour.
- Make an appetizer tray with roasted almonds, dried fruit, and low-fat cheeses.

Artichokes

2 heart-healthy reasons to eat your artichokes

Is it a vegetable? Is it a fruit? Actually, it's a thistle, and it's packed with good-for-you nutrition. An American favorite since the 18th century — George Washington and Thomas Jefferson were both fans — the globe artichoke is highly regarded for its healing abilities. From digestive woes to heart health, this delicious thistle has something for everyone. Read on to find out how this odd-looking prickly plant can keep your ticker fine-tuned.

Lower your blood pressure with fiber and potassium.
Researchers studied over 200 volunteers assigned to different diets. After three months, those who agreed to stick to a high-fiber menu with lots of whole-grain foods, noted a significant drop in blood pressure. High fiber was the key.

But whole grains aren't the only way to go. One medium globe artichoke provides 10 grams of fiber, helping you close in on that recommended goal of 25 to 35 grams per day.

And artichoke's potassium goes arm-in-arm with lower blood pressure. Experts say increasing the potassium in your diet is as important for healthy blood pressure as keeping tabs on your sodium. Just one fresh medium artichoke can supply you with 10 percent of the potassium you need every day.

Take aim at cholesterol with artichoke's secret weapon.
Artichoke leaf extract (ALE) is a supplement made from the long bottom leaves of the plant. Here much of the healthy

stuff, like natural plant chemicals called polyphenols, is found in abundance. With ALE, you get all the artichoke goodness in a very concentrated form.

One of these polyphenols, cynarin — pronounced "sigh-na-rin" — is credited with improving cholesterol levels in a study of over 140 people. After taking ALE for six weeks, their bad (LDL) cholesterol dropped by 23 percent. More good news? Their total cholesterol numbers decreased by nearly 20 percent. And additional research shows that artichoke leaf extract is effective for raising good HDL cholesterol, too.

In the fight against heart disease, the humble artichoke stands out as a big winner.

Globe or Jerusalem: what's the difference?

They both go by the name "artichoke," but they couldn't be more different. From the globe's tender, tasty leaves to the Jerusalem's crunchy root, these plants have little in common. Even their origins can be traced to opposite sides of the world. The globe hails from the sunny Mediterranean region, while the gnarly root of the Jerusalem artichoke, also known as a sunchoke, got its start in North America.

Their nutrients differ, too. The globe artichoke is rich in vitamin K , folate, and fiber, but the Jerusalem variety is packed with iron and potassium.

And the Jerusalem is easier to prepare. Experts recommend cooking it just like you would a potato. Try it roasted, baked, boiled, with the skin or without. Most surprising? You can even eat it raw.

Kitchen know-how: enjoy the perfect artichoke

Their appearance is a little daunting. All those spiky leaves, the tough stem. And what's up with that fuzzy choke part? Don't be overwhelmed. Here's a handy guide to help you select, prepare, and eat this odd-looking thistle.

Start by choosing an artichoke that's compact but feels heavy for its size. Look for leaves that are tight and bright green. If they are dried out or feathery, or if they bend easily — instead of snapping off crisply — pick another artichoke. That one's past its prime.

To prepare, cut off the top third of the artichoke and remove the tough outer leaves. Then simmer it in boiling water with lemon juice for about thirty minutes, or until a sharp knife easily cuts through its base.

At the store, hold the artichoke to your ear and give it a good squeeze. Hear that squeak? That means it's fresh. As artichokes age, their leaves lose that crispness. Squeaky leaves are a sign that it's straight from the farm.

Remember to use a stainless steel, enamel, or glass pan for cooking. Cookware made from copper, cast iron, or aluminum might cause your artichokes to discolor. And here's a tip the pros know. Artichokes float. Place a small lid over your artichokes in the pot to keep them submerged while they cook.

Now that you've selected and prepared your artichoke, it's time to dig in and savor the deliciousness. But just how do you do that? Start with the leaves. Pull one off and dip it in your favorite sauce. Then gently scrape the leaf through your teeth to remove the tasty treat at the base. Discard the remains. Continue one by one until you've finished off all the leaves.

Next, spoon out the fuzzy center called the choke. Don't eat this part, just throw it away. But the bottom — the heart — is delicious. Cut it into small pieces and enjoy.

Artichokes fight 3 deadly cancers

Breast cancer. Skin cancer. Pancreatic cancer. Each one a terrible disease. But researchers say you can up your protection against all three with powerful compounds found in artichokes.

Block breast cancer cell growth. Polyphenols are natural plant chemicals that can slow down or even stop the progress of diseases like cancer. Use them to hit breast cancer hard with a one-two artichoke punch.

- First, hit it high. Scientists discovered high doses of artichoke extract (AE) caused breast cancer cells to die.

- Next, hit it low. Long-term, low doses of AE prevented breast cancer cells from growing and dividing.

Researchers agree that artichokes' polyphenols may be key to the development of new, innovative therapies in the fight against breast cancer.

> Those tender green artichoke leaves left on your plate look innocent enough. What damage could they possibly do to your garbage disposal? Plenty. Artichoke fibers can get caught in the inner workings of your disposal, causing it to shut down — perhaps for good. Toss them in a compost bin instead.

Safeguard your skin with artichoke's silymarin. This powerful artichoke compound has anti-inflammatory, antioxidant, and anti-cancer properties. That's a lot of "anti" power packed into one small plant.

Usually taken as a capsule or tablet, silymarin triggers apoptosis in melanoma cells. In other words, it causes them to die. And research even suggests that adding silymarin to sunscreen and other skin products might prove to be one easy, all-natural way to protect against sun damage from ultraviolet A rays.

Dynamic duo offers promise against pancreatic cancer. Apigenin and luteolin. Think of them as superheroes, ready to wage war on pancreatic cancer — the fourth leading cause of cancer-related deaths.

Researchers at the University of Illinois discovered these two flavonoids kill pancreatic cancer cells in the lab by blocking a necessary enzyme. They hope someday to design a drug that would raise blood levels of the flavonoids high enough to achieve the same results in pancreatic cancer patients. "If you eat a lot of fruits and vegetables throughout your life, you'll have chronic exposure to these bioactive flavonoids," says study author Elvira de Mejia, "which would certainly help to reduce the risk of cancer."

Hankering for a hint of something sweet? Try this. Eat an artichoke, sip some water, and — like magic — you'll taste a burst of sweetness. Except it's not magic. When you chew artichokes, a natural chemical called cynarin blocks your tongue's sweet receptors. Drink water, and the cynarin washes away, leaving behind that sugary sensation. No magic — just sweet science.

ALE tackles tummy troubles

It's more than a tummy ache. There's belching, nausea, and bloating. You feel full too fast when you're eating a meal. And who can forget the stomach pain? Your doctor says you have functional dyspepsia, a condition that affects up to one-third of adults.

In a German study, half a group of people with functional dyspepsia took 320 milligrams of artichoke leaf extract (ALE) three times a day for six weeks. The other half took a placebo pill. When all was said and done, 85 percent of those taking ALE reported marked improvement in their stomach symptoms.

Researchers think ALE stimulates the flow of bile, a digestive fluid made in your liver and stored in your gallbladder. Bile's job is to help absorb fats and certain vitamins. Without enough, you can feel all kinds of digestive woes. ALE helps bile get food moving quickly though your system, which cuts down on symptoms like fullness and bloating. A welcome relief for the discomforts of dyspepsia.

Choose frozen over fresh for no-fuss meals

You're craving artichokes for dinner, but it's a busy weeknight. Who has time for all that prep work? Here's an alternative that gets to the heart of the problem — go for frozen instead of fresh.

Available in boxes or bags, frozen artichokes come cleaned, trimmed, and cooked. And they don't have any of the strong flavors you often find in canned or jarred varieties.

Start by thawing them completely and draining off any excess water. Next, give them a good squeeze, dry them thoroughly with paper towels, and they're ready for your recipe.

Compared to fresh, frozen artichoke hearts contain slightly fewer nutrients, but you may decide the convenience is worth it. Especially when you taste that delicious artichoke flavor in your favorite quick-as-a-wink weeknight supper.

Baking soda

Get back to basics and beat heartburn

Have you ever had heartburn so bad you can hear the flames crackling inside your chest? You'll do anything to cool the fire. Well, here's the good news. Relief is just inside your pantry.

Heartburn happens when your lower esophageal sphincter — the barrier between your esophagus and stomach — doesn't close properly. Stomach acid splashes into your esophagus and triggers a painful, burning sensation in your chest and throat.

That's where baking soda comes in. Chemically, it's a base, which just means it's the opposite of an acid. And when you mix an acid and a base, voilà, they cancel each other out. Using baking soda this way might seem odd, but it's surprisingly natural. Your pancreas produces the same active chemical that's in baking soda, sodium bicarbonate, to protect your intestines from stomach acid.

To treat your heartburn, stir half a teaspoon of baking soda into a cup of water. Drink this every two hours, or until you feel better. Just don't use this treatment for long-term heartburn — symptoms that last more than two weeks — since baking soda can have a toxic effect if you take it too often.

And remember, you'll get a whopping amount of salt in every dose. That half a teaspoon of baking soda contains over 600 milligrams of sodium.

Pepper protection: simple trick turns down the heat

Eating and cooking with hot peppers is always a gamble. Sometimes, they're packed with flavor and just a little bit of heat. But all too often, they set your mouth and fingers on fire. Fortunately, you don't have to suffer through the pain. This simple recipe will put out the blaze in no time. Mix together:

- 1/8 teaspoon baking soda

- 1 tablespoon water

- 1 tablespoon hydrogen peroxide

Hydrogen peroxide neutralizes capsaicin, the compound that gives hot peppers their painful burn. And adding a bit of baking soda makes it work even better.

Use this mixture to wash your hands after chopping hot peppers. You can also swish it as a mouthwash to cool the burn, but be careful not to swallow.

The complete kitchen cleaning kit — all for under $10

Do you really need a stockpile of supplies to wipe up every kitchen smudge and stain? Most people spend over $200 a year on cleaning products. But with a little know-how you can get five cleaning products to do it all — for less than $10. They'll take on messes even better than name-brand options.

Make your sinks sparkle and battle grease stains with baking soda. A 16-ounce box of baking soda won't set you back more than $0.75, and yet it's the best way to tackle tough stains on your sink. All you need to do is make a paste with equal parts baking soda and water and start scrubbing away. After a quick rinse your basin will look like new.

Baking soda is also a great way to clean that sticky residue left on baking pans. While the pan is still warm, throw some baking soda on the oily gunk. As it cools, the baking soda will soak up all the grease.

Vanquish dishwasher funk with vinegar. A half gallon of plain white vinegar only costs about $1.60, and it's just as good — if not better — than all those expensive cleaning products.

And while you may think vinegar, lemonade, and baking soda are an unlikely combination, these three actually have some amazing uses. They'll do wonders for one of the toughest-to-clean appliances in your kitchen — the dishwasher.

To get rid of stains and smells, empty your dishwasher, and work your way through these three steps.

1. Fill a dishwasher-safe cup with vinegar and place in the top rack. Run a hot wash cycle to loosen the stains and get to work on that musty smell.

2. Next run a wash cycle with powdered lemonade instead of soap. The citric acid and lemony scent will really freshen things up.

3. To further deodorize and blast away stains, sprinkle a good handful of baking soda in the bottom of your dishwasher and run it again on the hottest cycle.

Bleach banishes dangerous bacteria. Believe it or not, a gallon of bleach is the most expensive cleaning supply you'll ever need. And it only costs $3.

When you're going up against food-borne bacteria, you need to call on the big guns. Wiping down your countertops or cutting boards with a bit of bleach will keep your kitchen bacteria-free. Just make sure you:

- dilute it — two tablespoons to every quart of water should do.

- don't use on certain surfaces, like granite.

- never, ever mix bleach with other cleaners.

Salt scrubs away stuck-on food. A box of salt belongs in every kitchen, but not because you'll need it to season your food. For less than $1, you'll have one of the best solutions for caked-on messes.

If you can't get dried food off of your pots and pans, mix three tablespoons of salt with enough warm water to cover the food. Let it soak for a few hours and everything should scrape right off.

Hydrogen peroxide can save your scratched plates. It's a must for any first aid-kit, but hydrogen peroxide is not only for scraped elbows and knees.

Pick up a bottle for about a dollar, and use it to remove scratches from your white dishes. Just make a paste out of 1 teaspoon hydrogen peroxide and 2 tablespoons baking soda. Rub the paste all over your plates and let them sit for 12 hours. When you rinse them off, they'll look better than the day you bought them.

Bargain bonanza — 9 ways to save big at the supermarket

Swapping store-bought cleaners for baking soda can save you hundreds of dollars, but don't let the savings stop there. Generic baking soda is just as good as the name-brand stuff, and it's much cheaper. The same goes for most other pantry staples, too. If you buy the right brands and follow these tips, you can trim $50 to $150 a month off your grocery bill — without cutting back on food.

- Make sure the price is right. Learn how much common items usually cost, so you know a good deal when you see it. Pay attention to the price per unit to more effectively compare prices.

- Bend for bargains. Stores put the most popular and expensive items at eye level. Stoop to check out the bottom shelves and get the best deals.

- Time it right. Shop on Tuesdays or Wednesdays, when super-markets run most of their specials and stores are less crowded.

- Scale back. Ask the store to break up bunches of produce so you can buy a smaller amount. Don't pay for more than you will eat.

- Walk past gimmicks. Supermarkets display items at the ends of aisles to make you think they are a special deal. They're usually not.

- Shop seasonally. When markets have an abundance of certain foods, prices drop.

- Get inside tips. Chat with your grocers. You may find out about special deals from stocking clerks, butchers, and store managers.

- Double-check at checkout. Watch the register and check receipts. Mistakes can happen. A checker may scan an item twice or the sale price may not ring up.

Browning onions? This kitchen hack will save you time

There's no way around it — browning onions is a pain. Doing it right means standing over a stove, sometimes for hours, stirring at low heat, and hoping you don't burn anything. But if you add a bit of baking soda, you'll have perfectly caramelized onions in minutes.

It sounds strange, but there's science behind this magic trick. When food cooks, it goes through a series of chemical reactions. Adding a weak base, like baking soda, speeds up these reactions and literally cooks your food faster.

Be careful not to add too much baking soda, however, because it can change the flavor of your onions. Aim for around one-fourth teaspoon per pound of onions — although if you don't notice a taste difference, feel free to use a touch more.

Pamper your skin without sacrificing your wallet

Taking care of your skin is important, but all those store-bought products are hard on your bank account. If you want a little pampering without spending hundreds, just open up your pantry. A bit of baking soda will make you glow — and it will only set you back a few cents.

Take the natural path to smoother skin. No, you don't have to spend a fortune on fancy exfoliators to get a soft, smooth complexion. Instead mix 2 tablespoons of water and 1 tablespoon of baking soda into a paste and gently rub in small circles on your face. Rinse clean and pat dry.

If you have fragile or particularly sensitive skin, test on a small patch first to see if this is too abrasive for you.

Raid the pantry to soothe your sunburn. The tops of your feet. The tips of your ears. Your neck. Where did you last fail to apply sunscreen? And now you're dealing with a fiery red, oh-so tender burn.

Using the same 2-1 ratio, make a paste out of water and baking soda. Gently pat it onto those burned spots, let sit for a few minutes, and rinse off with cool water.

You can also mix a cup of baking soda into a lukewarm bath to soak away the itch and pain. Let your skin air-dry and you'll feel better in no time.

The all-natural way to keep bugs at bay

Nobody wants to find creepy, crawly insects in their kitchen. But you also don't want to spread dangerous chemicals around the house — especially if you have pets or small children. For a safer way to keep the bugs away, reach for your baking soda.

Mix together equal parts baking soda and sugar and sprinkle around the corners of your kitchen. Or fill small dishes or jar lids with the mixture and set inside cabinets. Bugs will be attracted to the sweet taste of sugar, but they won't be able to digest the baking soda.

Barley

Whole-grain goodness for a longer life

Decisions, decisions. A lean waist with less belly fat or a healthier heart. If you had to pick, which would you choose? Turns out this is a trick question. Whole-grain barley, a cheap, delicious, easy-to-find food, gives you both.

Bring on the barley for a trimmer middle. Here's a frightening fact. Men and women with large waists die younger, usually from heart disease, respiratory problems, or cancer, compared to those with slimmer middles.

Researchers studied more than 650,000 people over 15 years, and their findings were stunning. For every extra two inches of belly fat, the chance of death went up 7 percent in men, and a scary 9 percent in women.

So what's a body to do? Add more whole grains like barley to your diet. A Japanese study gave 44 men either rice or a barley-rice mixture to add to their meals for 12 weeks. When the study ended, researchers found the barley group had less visceral fat — the deep-in-the-belly kind that can lead to heart disease — and slimmer waists.

Whole-grain barley lowers two kinds of cholesterol. Bad cholesterol sky-high? Barley's fiber can help get those numbers down. Studies show fiber — like the kind in barley — effectively shrinks bad LDL cholesterol as well as non-HDL cholesterol,

which is your total cholesterol minus your good HDL cholesterol. And that's great news for your heart.

But here's the bad news. Research shows 90 percent of Americans
don't get close to the recommended amount of daily fiber in
their diet — 25 grams for women and 38 grams for men. In
fact, the average American gets about 15 grams per day.
Sometimes even less.

You can lower your non-HDL and your LDL cholesterol simply
by including more whole-grain fiber like barley in your menu.

U.S. federal regulations support the recommendation that eating 3 grams or more per day of barley's soluble fiber will reduce
your risk of heart disease. Generally, one cup of cooked pearl
barley gives you 2.5 grams of soluble fiber.

The facts are plain and simple. Want to live longer? Eat more
whole grains like barley.

Barley and beans, food fit for a gladiator

Roman gladiators were nicknamed "hordearii" — barley
men — and for good reason, researchers discovered, when
they unearthed a gladiator graveyard near the ancient city
of Ephesus, now in modern Turkey.

When the bones of 60 of these fierce fighters were examined, scientists determined the gladiator diet consisted of
beans, barley, and just a little animal protein.

Although this high-carb diet made the battlers a bit pudgy,
the excess padding came in handy. Experts think it pro-
vided the combatants with an extra layer of protection that
shielded them from deep cuts, blood vessel wounds, and
nerve injuries during battle.

Stave off snack attacks with barley's filling fiber

Barley is brimming with viscous fiber. What's viscous, you ask? Most dictionaries define it as "a substance that's thick, gelatinous, or gummy." Doesn't sound very appetizing, does it? But maybe you'll find it more appealing when you realize that viscous fiber — also known as soluble fiber — can help you beat back those calorie-packed nighttime cravings.

Check your appetite at the door. The refrigerator door, that is. A study in *The Journal of Nutrition* found people who ate barley bread during an evening meal felt fuller than those who ate refined grains, like white wheat bread. And if you feel full, you're less likely to cave to those after-supper cravings.

Viscous fiber is found in barley and many other foods like fresh apples, oats, mushrooms, and baked beans. As this fiber passes through your digestive system, the liquids in your stomach and intestines mix it into a thick gel. That's where the "gummy" part comes in. This gel stays in your system where it helps block your appetite for up to two more meals. Starting to like the sound of this?

Celiac disease is an autoimmune disorder where eating foods containing gluten — a protein found in wheat, rye, barley, and certain other grains — can damage your small intestine. If you have been diagnosed with celiac disease, check labels for hidden gluten on processed foods like pastas, pastries, cereals, and even your favorite croutons. Find out more online at *celiac.org*.

Add fiber to your diet — a little at a time. It may be tempting to go full speed ahead on the barley bandwagon, but it's best to proceed slowly. Adding too much fiber too fast can bring on digestive issues like abdominal cramps, bloating, diarrhea, and gas.

Start off by introducing high-fiber whole grains to your menu several times a week. Continue to up your intake of viscous fiber for two or three weeks until you reach your target goal — a little over 9 grams of soluble fiber per day for men, and 6 daily grams for women.

And don't forget to hydrate. Six to eight glasses of water every day will help your body process that fiber. So will some regular exercise.

Barley water: from Wimbledon with love

Refreshing barley water makes a cool summertime treat. Just ask the folks at Wimbledon, London, site of the oldest and most famous tennis tournament in the world. And where Robinson's Barley Water has been the official beverage of the strawberries-and-cream crowd since 1935.

It all began when a Robinson's employee combined the company's barley crystals — made from barley and other grains — with lemon juice, sugar, and water to create a delicious, hydrating drink for the tennis players.

No need to jet to London for a sample, though. Make it yourself with this simple recipe.

Place the peel and juice of two lemons in a 3-quart pitcher. Set aside. In a medium saucepan, combine 2 quarts water and 1 cup uncooked hulled barley. Bring to a boil, cover, and simmer for 30 minutes. Pour through a fine-mesh strainer into your pitcher. (Save the cooked barley to toss into your favorite soup or casserole.) Stir in 1/4 cup honey. Refrigerate.

Build better bones with barley's nutrients

Sing along! Cranium, scapula, patella, phalanges. These lyrics don't sound familiar? You might know them better as "head, shoulders, knees, and toes." Four of barley's special nutrients help keep all your bones strong and healthy — from your cranium to your phalanges — no matter what you call them.

* Calcium. Bet you're already familiar with this bone-healthy powerhouse. Got milk, right? But there are other sources of calcium, too. A cup of cooked pearl barley, for example, provides 2 percent of your recommended daily value.

* Magnesium. When it teams up with calcium and other minerals, your bones are in for a real boost. To get 9 percent of your recommended daily value of magnesium, dig into a cup of cooked pearl barley.

* Zinc. This mighty mineral keeps your body humming along in many ways, from healing wounds to fighting off viruses. But you also need zinc to absorb calcium. How much? Recommended intake for men is 11 milligrams (mg) and 8 mg for women. A cup of cooked pearl barley supplies your bones with 1.3 mg of zinc.

* Manganese. A true nutritional superstar, manganese is crucial for lots of body processes, from building healthy bones to promoting normal brain function. Experts estimate that up to 37 percent of Americans don't get the recommended amount of manganese — 1.8 mg for women and 2.3 mg for men. Good to know one cup of cooked pearl barley provides you with a whopping 20 percent of your daily requirement.

Pearl or hulled? Go with the grain that's right for you

Ready to add some barley to your diet, but bewildered by which kind to buy? Not sure exactly how to cook it? Here's a barley primer to help you add this healthy grain to your menu. Pearls of barley wisdom, you might say.

When in doubt, choose pearl. You've found a recipe you're excited to try, but it doesn't tell you what kind of barley to use. Here's a tip — if the recipe doesn't specify, play it safe with pearl.

This type of barley has been polished or "pearled" to remove the tough outer hull. And even though pearl barley is not really a whole grain, it's healthier than other refined grains because its fiber is spread throughout the entire barley kernel, not just its outer layer.

Store uncooked barley in an airtight container in your refrigerator or freezer for up to six months. Cooked barley — pearl or hulled — will stay fresh for up to a week in the fridge, or up to six months in your freezer. Cook's tip — let barley come to room temperature before using.

You'll usually find it on your supermarket shelves, tucked in between the lentils and dried beans. It may be labeled as regular, medium, fine, or baby pearl, depending on how much the grain has been processed. And color counts, too. If the barley is lightly pearled, it will have a tan color. Heavily pearled, highly polished barley is white.

To cook pearl barley, bring 3 cups water to a boil. Add 1 cup pearl barley, and return to a boil. Reduce heat, cover, and simmer for 45 minutes, until the kernels are tender and the liquid is absorbed.

For whole-grain goodness, go with hulled. Also called barley groats or dehulled barley, hulled has a chewier texture and heartier flavor than pearl barley. Hulled barley is considered a whole grain because it has only the tough outer hull removed, leaving the rest of the kernel intact.

For best flavor and a shorter prep time, soak your hulled barley overnight — or at least for a few hours prior to cooking. When you're ready, add 1 cup grain to 3 cups boiling water in a medium saucepan. Cover and return to boil. Reduce heat to low, and cook for 50 to 55 minutes. You'll know it's ready when the amount of barley in your pot has tripled and it's soft, but chewy.

Hulled barley doesn't absorb as much liquid as pearl barley does, so you may have to pour off extra liquid at the end of the cooking time.

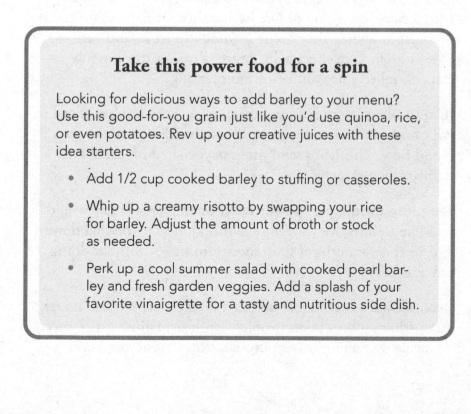

Take this power food for a spin

Looking for delicious ways to add barley to your menu? Use this good-for-you grain just like you'd use quinoa, rice, or even potatoes. Rev up your creative juices with these idea starters.

- Add 1/2 cup cooked barley to stuffing or casseroles.

- Whip up a creamy risotto by swapping your rice for barley. Adjust the amount of broth or stock as needed.

- Perk up a cool summer salad with cooked pearl barley and fresh garden veggies. Add a splash of your favorite vinaigrette for a tasty and nutritious side dish.

Beets

Supercharge your life with a crimson root

This up-and-coming sports drink bumps up your get-up-and-go, so you can exercise longer with less effort. No, it's not a sugar-laden or calorie-filled drink. The best beverage for improving workout performance is one you probably never think of — beet juice.

These root vegetables are packed with nitrates. Wait, nitrates are bad, right? Well, these compounds can be dangerous when added to processed foods like bacon and hot dogs. But they are not harmful when they occur naturally in fruits and veggies. The vitamin C in them helps prevent cancer-causing substances, called nitrosamines, from forming.

Instead, these nitrates create nitric oxide, which is beneficial to your body. Nitric oxide relaxes blood vessels and improves blood flow. This helps send more oxygenated blood to your hardworking muscles.

Plug into produce to power up your muscles. How would you like to improve your muscle function as if you had done two to three months of resistance training — without doing any exercise?

Beetroot juice may be the key, says a recent study. Two hours after drinking beet juice, people with heart failure experienced a 13-percent rise in power in muscles that extend the knee.

"A lot of daily activities are power-based — getting out of a chair, lifting groceries, climbing stairs. And they have a major impact on quality of life," says senior author Linda R. Peterson, MD. "Power is such an important predictor of how well people do, whether they have heart failure, cancer, or other conditions. In general, physically more powerful people live longer."

Raise your energy level with tasty roots. In addition to the power boost, studies show beetroot juice improves endurance and stamina, helping you exercise longer.

What about whole beets? They're cheaper and easier to find, and a recent study says they'll also do the trick. Volunteers ate a cup and a half of baked beets before running a 5K (3.1 miles) on a treadmill. They later repeated their performance after eating cranberry relish. Tests showed they ran 5 percent faster during the last mile after eating the beets compared to the cranberries. And they did it with less effort.

You may not have a 5K coming up any time soon, but if you want to add a little pep to your step, nitrate-rich beets may deliver what you need.

> Big beet eater? Don't be alarmed if you end up with red or pink urine. About one in 10 people experience this harmless condition known as beeturia. The culprits are betalains — pigments that give beets their deep red color. You can also find them added to other foods for color. Look for the combo "E162" in the ingredients list.

Root for a speedy recovery time. Want to bounce back faster from your workout? Not only will the nitrates in beets help, but so will a group of pigments known as betalains. These phytonu-trients work as antioxidants and anti-inflammatories to help you kiss muscle soreness and inflammation goodbye.

Out of 30 men performing strenuous exercise, those who drank 8.5 ounces of beetroot juice for three days afterward saw the best results, says a British study.

The juice sped up the time it took to erase the aches and pains that often accompany workout recovery. It's like a best friend who kicks out tiresome guests before they overstay their welcome.

And you don't have to be a gold-winning athlete to reap the benefits. "Those who exercise less tend to suffer from more muscle damage than those who exercise frequently," says study author Tom Clifford, Ph.D. "Beetroot would be more beneficial for your average Joe than someone who is more accustomed to exercise."

'Beet' high blood pressure

A daily glass of beetroot juice may be just what you need to control your blood pressure, says a study in *Hypertension*. The nitrates in beets relax your arteries and improve blood flow. Lower pressure means less risk for heart attack and stroke.

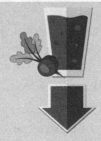

People who drank 8.5 oz a day for 4 weeks lowered blood pressure 8/4 mmHg.

Surprise! Beet greens are a healthy (and edible) treat

Beetroots give your meals a delicious red twist, but if you always throw out their green tops, you're missing out on another treat.

Beet greens have an impressive lineup of nutrients, including vitamin K, vitamin C, beta carotene, lutein, and zeaxanthin.

Snag the benefits by adding them to salads or blending them in smoothies. You can also soften these greens by lightly steaming or sautéing them with your favorite veggies.

Surefire ways to enjoy the benefits of beets

You may not live on a 60-acre beet farm like Dwight Schrute from the TV series "The Office," but getting your hands on these crimson roots isn't difficult. Here are some great ways to slip them into your diet.

- Savor the flavor in a juice. It may sound odd, but beet juice is quite the rage. Many stores sell bottles of beet juice, often called beetroot juice. If you can't find any at your local stores, you can get it online. The downside is the juice can be pricey.

- Save by juicing your own. To get beet juice without the big price tag, your best bet may be the produce aisle. Got a juicer or blender? Buy some fresh beets and make your own juice. You can even add other vegetables, like carrots, if you want to change up the taste.

- Eat them whole. Don't worry if you're not a fan of beet juice. Whole beets will still give you all the phytonutrients you need. Plus, you'll benefit from the fiber that's missing in the juice. Bake or roast whole beets as a side dish. Grate them into salads or cook them into soups. It's up to you. Studies show most cooking methods retain beets' beneficial antioxidants.

Can't 'beet' this way to boost memory

Where did you put your phone? When is your next doctor's appointment? And what was on your grocery list — the one your forgot at home? If your brain needs a little pick-me-up, turn to beets. Studies show they send oxygen straight to your head, replenishing your noggin where it needs it most.

The ravages of aging can interfere with blood flow to your brain. Sounds bad, doesn't it? It is. Decreased blood flow plays a part in dementia and problems with everyday brain activity like concentrating and learning new things.

This is where beets step in. Your body turns nitrates found in beets into nitric oxide, which can help open up blood vessels in your body, increasing blood flow.

"Nitric oxide is a really powerful molecule," says Jack Rejeski, a professor at Wake Forest University. "It goes to the areas of the body which are hypoxic, or needing oxygen, and the brain is a heavy feeder of oxygen in your body."

Rejeski co-authored a recent study that shows drinking beetroot juice before exercise fires up brain connections similar to those you see in younger adults.

His research team isn't the only one to prove beets can enhance the brains of older adults. Researchers in another study asked participants to eat a high-nitrate breakfast, which included 17 ounces of beet juice. Then they took an MRI of the subjects' brains to view blood flow. The test revealed better blood flow to regions of the brain commonly associated with mental decline.

So if you're needing a memory boost or sharper focus, power up on beets and other high-nitrate foods like Swiss chard, beet greens, spring greens, rhubarb, and arugula. They could give you a leg up on your daily activities, such as shopping, writing checks, and using appliances.

3 cheap fixes for messy red stains

Beets are fantastic, but that doesn't mean you want to wear them. Ward off stains and keep your kitchen clean by following these tips.

- The simplest solution is to wear rubber or latex gloves and layer your cutting board with wax paper. When you're done, just throw away the evidence.

- If you don't have those items, bring out the vegetable oil. Rub your beet-holding hand and cutting board with about half a teaspoon of oil, or spray with cooking spray. This will create a barrier so your skin and board won't soak up the juices.

- Already caught red-handed? Here's a popular natural solution. Wash your fuchsia fingers with lemon juice to remove the stains. If your hands feel dry after you rinse, follow with a moisturizer.

Beta glucans

Beta glucans offer a hat trick of health benefits

The best little fiber you've never heard of — beta glucan — is a complex sugar in the cell walls of plants like mushrooms, seaweed, and grains. In fact, two of your favorite whole grains, oats and barley, are chock-full of this fab fiber. Wouldn't it be great if you could eat delicious, inexpensive foods like these to lower your cholesterol, blood pressure, AND your blood sugar, instead of taking expensive drugs?

Guess what? Because of beta glucan, experts say you can.

Bring those cholesterol numbers down. Not all beta glucan has the same job, but the kind that's found in oats can help control your cholesterol.

It works by combining with water in your digestive system to form a thick gel. Once in the small intestine, this gel binds with fat-digesting bile acids your body makes out of cholesterol. Then the gel slowly sweeps the bile out of your system, sending your cholesterol — literally — down the drain. Once these bile acids are gone, your body gets busy making more out of the cholesterol you're storing in your liver. This helps drop your cholesterol numbers even lower.

Healthy blood pressure is within reach. Struggling to get your blood pressure below the 120/80 mark, as recommended by the American Heart Association? Beta glucan to the rescue.

In a three-month study, researchers found three servings a day of oat beta glucan effectively lowered blood pressure, especially in people who were extremely overweight. In fact, their systolic pressure — the top number — went down nearly six points, while their diastolic pressure — the bottom number — dropped a little over two points.

Tasty secret to steady blood sugar. Remember the thick beta glucan gel that lowered your cholesterol? Turns out it also keeps your glucose levels in check by slowing the way your body absorbs sugars.

The research results are simple and straightforward. Eat 4 grams of oat beta glucan every day to help control your blood sugar. Not hard to do. Just help yourself to 1 1/2 cups of tasty cooked oatmeal for breakfast. That's 3 grams of beta glucan right off the bat. Prefer barley to oats? Just 1 cup of cooked pearl barley provides you with 2.5 grams of beta glucan. A sweet way to start your day.

Bowled over: 4 surprising ways oats make your life easier

Think outside the bowl with these simple, "oat-standing" ideas that use uncooked, regular oats.

- Neutralize nasty fridge odors. Leave an uncovered bowl of oats in your refrigerator, let them work their magic, then discard.

- Oh, no. Someone spilled cooking oil in the middle of your kitchen floor. Pour your oat flakes on the puddle, and wait five minutes. Then give your floor a thorough sweep.

- No time to shampoo? Mix equal parts ground oatmeal and baking soda. Work the mixture into your dry roots, and then brush it out. Presto! Oil and dirt vanish.

- Cure the grandkids' rainy day blues with oat play dough. Combine 4 cups oats with 2 cups flour and 2 cups water. Stir. Makes enough for two artistic little ones, and the dough will stay soft for hours.

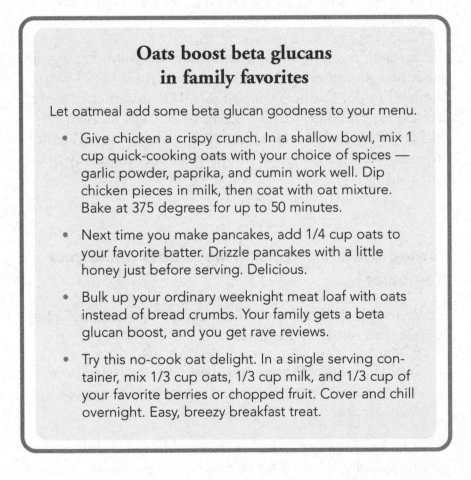

Oats boost beta glucans in family favorites

Let oatmeal add some beta glucan goodness to your menu.

- Give chicken a crispy crunch. In a shallow bowl, mix 1 cup quick-cooking oats with your choice of spices — garlic powder, paprika, and cumin work well. Dip chicken pieces in milk, then coat with oat mixture. Bake at 375 degrees for up to 50 minutes.

- Next time you make pancakes, add 1/4 cup oats to your favorite batter. Drizzle pancakes with a little honey just before serving. Delicious.

- Bulk up your ordinary weeknight meat loaf with oats instead of bread crumbs. Your family gets a beta glucan boost, and you get rave reviews.

- Try this no-cook oat delight. In a single serving container, mix 1/3 cup oats, 1/3 cup milk, and 1/3 cup of your favorite berries or chopped fruit. Cover and chill overnight. Easy, breezy breakfast treat.

Switch off diabetes and heart disease with this little button

They may be cute as a button, but these mushrooms are tough as nails when it comes to fighting heart disease and diabetes. Tip your cap to the simple button mushroom, a powerhouse of vitamins and fiber.

Button mushrooms, scientifically known as *Agaricus bisporus*, don't get the oohs and aahs afforded their cousins, the much more exotic-sounding creminis and portobellos. But they should. Good old plain buttons — found at your local grocers — are full of beta glucan fiber and nutrients like vitamin D, riboflavin, niacin, folate, and polyphenols.

- An Australian study found these feisty fungi can lower your LDL and total cholesterol, which protects you from heart disease.

- Studies also show the beta glucans can lower blood sugar and insulin levels after a meal by slowing the delivery of glucose into your bloodstream.

Cherry-pick your buttons at the grocery store. Unless you're an expert, don't eat mushrooms you find in the wild. Poisonous varieties look very similar to the edible kind, and cooking does not get rid of the poison.

At the market, choose mushrooms that are firm and have a nice even color. They should be dry to the touch, too. Pass by the mushrooms that look withered, slimy, or bruised. And if they're not pre-wrapped, give the mushrooms a good sniff. You should notice an earthy, pleasing aroma.

Chef's tip — if you're not too particular about their appearance, older mushrooms may actually give your dish a richer flavor. Just be sure to use them as soon as possible.

Don't lose your buttons — store them the right way. Too much air, and they dry out. Too tightly wrapped, and they get soggy. What can you do to keep them fresh?

Try this. Place your mushrooms in a loosely closed paper bag and store them in the main compartment of your refrigerator.

If you buy your mushrooms shrink-wrapped, just pop them in the fridge as is. They'll be good to go for up to one week. Cooked mushrooms are freezable, for even longer storage.

Aztec delicacy wows fiber-loving gourmets

Straight from the pre-Columbian cultures of Mexico, huitlacoche (weet-la-KOH-chay) is all the rage at fine-dining establishments around the world. Commonly known as corn smut — but also tagged "Mexican truffle" — huitlacoche is a mushroom-like fungus that grows on sweet corn.

Despite its unappetizing monikers, corn smut is rich in protein and its fiber can go toe-to-toe with oats. In fact, 2 to 8 percent of oat's whole grain is made up of beta glucan, while the amount of beta glucan in huitlacoche can go as high as 12 percent.

So are you adventurous enough to give it a try? Look for huitlacoche jarred, canned, or frozen at farmer's markets and Mexican grocery stores. Then enjoy its smoky, earthy flavor, with a taste like mushrooms mixed with corn. Simply spoon some over poached eggs or add to your favorite quesadilla. Olé!

These mushrooms help your body outsmart cancer

You've heard of Spiderman, Batman, and the Terminator, but how about the Immunomodulator? The name fits right in, doesn't it? So does its superpower. Beta glucan is known as an immunomodulator because it makes your immune system smarter and better equipped to fight off cancer.

- Certain kinds of beta glucan, like those in some mushrooms, can activate cancer-fighting cells called macrophages. These work like Pac-Man, ingesting and destroying cancer invaders.

- Beta glucan triggers your body to release cytokines, chemicals that help immune cells communicate with each other as they battle cancer cells. This makes your immune system much more efficient.

- And beta glucan fires up your body's lymphocytes, white blood cells that attach themselves to tumors or viruses and then release chemicals to destroy them.

Your body can't produce beta glucan on its own, so you have to get it from supplements or the foods you eat. Fancy an exotic fungus for dinner? Excellent choice. These mushrooms from around the world are rich sources of cancer-kicking beta glucan.

Shiitake mushrooms contain lentinan, a beta glucan which scientists believe may slow tumor growth. And researchers think lentinan may also extend the survival rate of people with stomach, colorectal, pancreatic, and liver cancers. Buy shiitakes dried or fresh at local markets and online.

Agaricus mushrooms, aka sun mushrooms, are grown in Brazil and Japan. Experts think the beta glucan in these mushrooms possess anti-tumor properties. And one study showed agaricus extract improved the quality of life for women with gynecological cancers. You can purchase agaricus extract at health food stores and online.

Chaga mushrooms from Russia are used in folk remedies across northern Europe. In laboratory and animal studies, researchers found evidence of compounds that can kill cancer cells and rev up your immune system. Chaga mushrooms taste very bitter, but you can buy them dried, as a capsule, or in tea bags.

Oyster mushrooms contain pleuran, another anti-tumor beta glucan, that increased cancer survival rates in animal studies. Pick up fresh, dried, or canned oyster mushrooms at whole food stores and online.

Boost your health, 1 spoonful at a time

Nutritional yeast. Its name doesn't exactly rev up your taste buds, does it? And it's not so great to look at either. In fact, critics compare its appearance to fish food. Ugh. But don't turn the page just yet. You won't want to miss out on the amazing health benefits found in this beta glucan-packed superfood.

Amp up your vim and vigor. Nutritional yeast, also known as "nooch," is an excellent source of nutrients. For example, just one tablespoon of Bragg's Nutritional Yeast Seasoning — sold at Whole Foods Markets and online — contains 3 grams of protein, 1 gram of fiber, and staggering amounts of B vitamins. Brands can vary, so be sure to read labels carefully.

Shake it like Parmesan. Devotees of nutritional yeast say its taste is a mix of nutty goodness and cheesy deliciousness. They describe it as "umami" — one of the five flavors humans taste, along with salty, sweet, bitter, and sour — and it means "a pleasant, savory taste." Think brothy or meaty.

Ready to give it a try? Start small. Sprinkle a little on your popcorn. Stir some into your next pot of soup. Shake a bit on your favorite pasta, and enjoy this healthful alternative to fatty Parmesan.

All yeasts are not the same. Nutritional yeast is grown, usually on molasses. It's harvested, heated, and dried — a process that deactivates the yeast. So just to be clear, this is not the kind you see in the baking aisle at the grocery store. That's baker's yeast, or active dry yeast. You use it to make baked goods, since it's still alive. Don't use this instead of nutritional yeast. You'll end up with an unappealing foamy mess.

> Just a spoonful a day stops the common cold dead in its tracks. Studies show nutritional yeast's beta glucan lowered the incidence of respiratory infection by up to 25 percent. And it could reduce cold-related sleeping troubles if you do get sick. So go ahead and feed your cold. Nutritional yeast, that is.

And another kind of yeast — brewer's yeast — is a very bitter byproduct of beer making. Don't substitute this for nutritional yeast, either. You won't be happy with the results.

Here's a storage tip. To preserve the B vitamins in nutritional yeast, keep it in a tightly lidded, dark glass or ceramic container. As long as the yeast stays dry, it can last for up to two years.

Bilberry extract

Powerful nutrients keep you looking sharp

Bilberries sound like they belong in a Dr. Seuss book. But unlike green eggs and ham, these tiny European berries are a real-life superfood. A close relative of the blueberry, they pack a mean nutritional punch.

But there's a little problem — bilberries are notoriously difficult to track down. Because they are mostly harvested from wild berry patches in places like Scotland, Norway, Sweden, and Finland, you probably won't see these fruits at your local grocery store. Fortunately, bilberry extracts and supplements are much easier to find. That means getting all the wonderful nutrients in these tart treats is a breeze — and you don't even need to take a trip across the pond.

Use natural compounds to brighten your vision. Bilberries are one of the best berries you can eat to protect your vision because they are chock-full of anthocyanins, plant chemicals that give fruits their dark blue and red colors. In fact, bilberries contain 15 natural anthocyanins, more than any other berry. And most of these reach your eye or retina intact, ready to help prevent vision loss.

Experts explain it this way. Over time, chronic inflammation and stress chip away at the sensitive cells in your eyes. The damage to these cells can affect your body's ability to produce rhopodsin, which is a pigment that improves your night vision and helps your eyes adapt to changing light. Numerous studies show low levels of rhopodsin cause vision problems and eye diseases, like age-related macular degeneration, glaucoma, and cataracts.

And that's where anthocyanins come in. In a Japanese study, mice treated with bilberry extracts containing about 39 percent anthocyanins had more rhodopsin in their eyes.

Iron-clad protection for your peepers. Too much heavy metal as a music choice can damage your hearing. But you probably didn't know heavy metal can cause you to lose your vision, too. Iron — a common mineral — might be the reason behind your fading eyesight. While your body needs some of this nutrient, excess iron damages the sensitive cells in your eyes.

But berry anthocyanins can save the day. They shield your vision from long-lasting injury by creating a protective barrier, which keeps your eyes from absorbing high doses of iron.

Get the berry best relief for your gut

Living with inflammatory bowel disease is like walking through a minefield — you're always tiptoeing around triggers and hoping nothing sets off a flare-up. But now, relief is on the horizon. Bilberry extracts might hold the secret to letting you regain control of your gut.

Experts still aren't quite sure what causes the two most common inflammatory bowel diseases, Crohn's disease and ulcerative colitis (UC), but the leading theories all point to the immune system. Your body's own defenses sometimes turn against you, causing chronic inflammation and painful bleeding in your intestinal tract.

Because of their powerful anti-inflammatory compounds, berry extracts are a popular treatment for these debilitating diseases. Anthocyanins are the key to berry's super powers. And if you want to get more of these miraculous chemicals, bilberry extracts are your best bet.

In a new study, Swiss researchers set out to discover just how these compounds work. They treated a small group of patients suffering from UC with an anthocyanin-rich bilberry extract. After six weeks, their levels of intestinal inflammation were drastically improved.

Experts think it's because bilberries help tame your immune system. The anthocyanins actually prevent messenger cells, called cytokines, from telling your body to attack itself.

The study's authors admit there's still a lot they don't know about bilberries, but the extracts may help if you're suffering from inflammatory bowel disease. Just make sure you talk to your doctor before trying any new supplements.

Take a leaf out of the history books to defeat diabetes

When you're picking berries, you probably don't think to grab a handful of leaves, too. But this might just change your mind. Long before doctors prescribed pills for diabetes, Europeans used bilberry leaves as powerful home remedies. In fact, people still brew them into teas to treat their symptoms. Now, researchers are starting to understand why bilberry leaves and their extracts deserve a spot in your medicine cabinet.

Bilberry leaves are loaded with powerful antioxidants and natural compounds that make them perfect for warding off diabetes.

Making them into extracts concentrates their powers —
and now a new study is starting to uncover just how these
chemicals work.

The antioxidants hidden in bilberry leaves target two specific
enzymes that help your body digest carbohydrates. Essentially,
they keep your body from absorbing too much sugar, much like
prescription diabetes drugs.

Bilberry leaf extracts are available at most local markets and
online. Put a few drops of the extract into warm water and
drink daily. Diabetes is a serious condition, so talk to your
doctor before trying this — especially if you are already taking
prescription medications.

Supplement shopping — 2 tricks to pick a winner

For every truly great supplement on the shelves, there's a
handful of bad ones that overpromise and underdeliver. Here
are a couple of tricks and tips to keep you from wasting
your hard-earned cash on a bottle of duds.

- Get the best bang for your buck. Anthocyanins are
  what make bilberries so powerful, but some supplements skimp on their ingredients. When you're
  choosing a brand, make sure it's worth the money.
  So look for products labeled with either 25 percent
  anthocyanidins or 36 percent anthocyanosides.

- Track down the real deal. Bilberry extract can get
  expensive, so some manufactures cut corners by using
  fillers or fake bilberries, like huckleberry or Chinese
  bilberry. Look for extracts made from real European
  bilberries, which are known as *Vaccinium myrtillus*.

Cantaloupe

1 marvelous melon: sweet protection against 8 cancers

Cancer and cantaloupe? Seems those luscious melon balls do more than just look good in a fruit salad — they give you the nutrients you need to guard against a whopping eight different cancers.

That's what multiple studies show and it's all thanks to phyto-chemicals, natural compounds in fruits and vegetables that promote good health while battling a host of diseases.

When you bite into a cantaloupe wedge, you're getting a mouthful of specific phytochemicals called carotenoids. Researchers have discovered carotenoids, like beta carotene and lycopene, are antioxidants, those powerful cancer-crushers you've read about for years.

For starters, carotenoids boost the cells that strengthen your immune system. They also block tumor growth, destroy cancer cells, and stop cancer cells from growing and spreading.

Research shows carotenoids not only lower the risk of breast cancer recurrence but minimize your chances of developing these cancers in the first place:

- breast
- cervical
- colon
- esophageal
- ovarian
- pancreatic
- prostate
- stomach

An impressive list, don't you think?

Wash away dangerous germs

Cantaloupes grow low to the ground where their rinds come in contact with all sorts of pests, chemicals, pesticides, and nasty little microorganisms like the ones that cause *Salmonella* and *Listeria*. These foodborne infections can make you feel like never getting out of bed again. In some cases, they have proven fatal.

In recent years, public health experts blamed tainted cantaloupes for the *Salmonella* and *Listeria* outbreaks that caused the deaths of close to 40 people in the U.S. What's a melon lover to do?

First, recognize that while these germs live on the outer shell of a cantaloupe, they can easily slide into the edible part when you slice one open. Then practice the following food safety guidelines so you can savor sweet cantaloupes free of worry.

> When you feel the pain and discomfort of heartburn, reach for fruit. But not just any fruit. Those high in natural acids like citrus, cranberries, and tomatoes will make your symptoms worse. Instead, cut open a cantaloupe, watermelon, or honeydew. These low-acid melons will cool the burn.

- Don't choose melons with dents, dark spots, or anything you think might be mold.

- Wash your hands with warm, soapy water.

- Wash and sanitize your knife and cutting board.

- Scrub the outside of the cantaloupe with a vegetable brush under cool tap water.

- Dry your melon thoroughly.

- Remove and discard the rind.

- Refrigerate melon pieces within two hours of cutting.

The inside scoop —
2 terrific timesaving tips

Break out the cheese slicer and ice cream scoop the next time you bring home a cantaloupe. These two essential tools will make preparing and serving your melon a whole lot easier.

Scoop out the seeds. Spooning the inner pulp out of a cantaloupe is like shoveling snow. You dig and dig, creating a big, slushy mess. Grab your ice cream scoop instead.

- Slice your melon in half.

- Take your ice cream scoop and remove the seeds in one clean swoop.

Easy-peasy rind removal. The best thing about cantaloupe is the juicy fruit on the inside. The worst thing — removing its thick, bumpy rind. Not anymore.

- After you clean away the seeds, cut your cantaloupe into wedges.

- Use a wire cheese slicer to smoothly peel off the rind.

Mighty mineral safeguards your heart

High blood pressure can be a real heartbreaker. Not only does it increase your chances of having a heart attack, it raises your risk of stroke, too. But just like love can mend a broken heart, cantaloupe can conquer out-of-control blood pressure, thanks to its high levels of potassium.

Scientists looked at 19 clinical trials on potassium and discovered in every single case, potassium supplements lowered both the systolic and diastolic numbers of blood pressure readings, important indicators of how much force your blood is exerting against your artery walls.

If that isn't enough, taking potassium also lowered the risk of stroke death by 40 percent, according to a 12-year study.

While most potassium trials involve supplements, experts agree the best way to get more of this powerful mineral is from food. And that's where cantaloupe comes in. One cup serves up 473 milligrams of potassium or 14 percent of the amount you need each day. That will do plenty to get your BP back on track.

> Did you know your body is made up of 60 percent water? And for good reason. You need liquids to regulate your temperature, lubricate your joints, and flush out waste, among other things. To replenish those oh-so-important fluids, eat cantaloupe. With a water content of 90 percent, this succulent melon will really get the job done.

Potassium benefits your heart because it:

- helps your body excrete harmful sodium.

- stimulates your heart muscle to beat regularly.

- increases the amount of urine you excrete which helps regulate the amount of fluid in your blood.

- raises nitric oxide levels which helps relax your arteries and improve blood flow.

- blocks free radicals.

- protects your blood vessels if you have high blood pressure due to salt sensitivity.

Welcome these 7 melon hacks

Want to enjoy cantaloupe's goodness to its fullest? Don't just chop it for fruit salads and smoothies. Give these surprising tips a try.

- Blend 1 1/2 tablespoons of the cantaloupe's pulp and seeds with a small banana and a tablespoon of raw honey. Massage onto your face, avoiding the eye area. Leave on for 10 to 15 minutes, and rinse with cool water.

- Whip up refreshing summery pops by puréeing cantaloupe with a pinch of sugar and a splash of lime juice. Pour into molds and freeze.

- Cook cubes on the grill kebab-style and dip in yogurt.

- Hang pieces of rind with a little flesh still on them near bird feeders or in your pet's birdcage. Your feathered friends will chirp, "Thank you."

- Roast cantaloupe seeds for about 10 minutes in a pan with a little oil and spices. A great golden, crispy snack.

- Chop the rind into chunks and toss into your compost pile.

- Purée 3 wedges of peeled cantaloupe with 1 tablespoon honey and 3 tablespoons cornmeal. Apply this moisturizing conditioner to wet hair for 10 minutes, then rinse thoroughly.

Watch out for allergy triggers

As much as you love cantaloupe, it may not be good for you if you have allergies. All because of something called Oral Allergy Syndrome (OAS). This is when your sensitivity to pollens and grasses causes a reaction to fruits, vegetables, and other plants with similar proteins.

Let's say you have an allergy to birch tree pollen. If you're like many, you may experience itchiness and swelling in your throat after eating an apple or celery. The same can happen to ragweed sufferers when they eat cantaloupe or other melons like honeydew and watermelon — especially during allergy season.

"Difficulty breathing and itchy rashes are signs to go to a board-certified allergist," says Dr. Joseph Leija, an allergist out of Illinois, "or, in extreme cases, straight to the emergency room."

Chicory root

Chicory gets to the root of heart health

It's been a popular health food since before there were, well, health foods — with roots all the way back to ancient Egypt, where it was cultivated more than 5,000 years ago. Eventually chicory branched out around the globe, even to far-off Greece. In fact, Greek physician, Galenus, nicknamed it "Friend of the Liver."

While Galenus was on to something, he just picked the wrong body part. He had no way of knowing chicory was full of natural plant chemicals called polyphenols — just what you need for a healthy heart. Turns out chicory helps keep clots from forming, so your blood flows smoothly.

A cup a day keeps the doctor away. In one study, volunteers drank about a cup of chicory coffee every day for a week. By the end of the week, their blood and plasma viscosity — how thick and sticky it is — was reduced significantly. And since this viscosity is used by doctors to detect inflammation and cardiac failure, that's pretty heartwarming news.

Give the credit to a plant polyphenol in chicory called caffeic acid, not to be confused with caffeine. Chicory is naturally caffeine-free.

> To make caffeine-free chicory coffee, bring 2 cups of water to a boil in a saucepan. Add 4 tablespoons of roasted, ground chicory root. Cover and simmer for 10 to 15 minutes. For a traditional New Orleans Café au Lait, combine equal parts hot chicory coffee and hot milk.

High cholesterol is history. A specific type of fiber found in chicory root, called inulin, lowers your bad LDL levels by binding with cholesterol particles in your digestive system and then moving them out of your body before you can absorb them.

To learn more about inulin and cholesterol, researchers asked people to eat a breakfast cereal fortified with 9 grams of inulin, or they could add a powdered form of the fiber — totaling 10 grams— to their beverages or meals. After four weeks, total and LDL cholesterol numbers went down, and the breakfast cereal folks saw their triglycerides drop a whopping 27 percent.

If Galenus knew then what you know now, he would have changed that nickname. "Friend of the Heart" has a nicer ring to it, don't you think?

Chicory leaf is a powerhouse of nutrition

The chicory plant is packed with nutritional clout, from its woody root to its purply-blue blooms. Just ask the Centers for Disease Control and Prevention, better known as the CDC. Experts there listed chicory as one of their top 10 powerhouse foods. To qualify, a 100-calorie serving had to provide an average of 10 percent or more of the daily recommended amount of 17 healthy nutrients.

Among the disease-fighting vitamins and minerals in chicory's leafy tops — vitamins A, C, and K, fiber, folate, and calcium.

A popular way to serve these mighty greens is to boil them until tender, drain, and then sauté quickly in olive oil and garlic.

Special fiber serves up a trio of health perks

Inulin is a type of fiber you'll find naturally in some plant foods
— including chicory root. And because inulin is so healthy,
cheap, and gives food a moist, creamy texture, manufacturers
also add it to lots of processed foods, from yogurt to energy
bars. Want some good news? The same stuff that gives ice
cream its smooth consistency also supports your bone health,
aids weight loss, and promotes a healthy digestive tract. What
more could you ask for?

Inulin makes stronger bones. In a yearlong study, researchers
discovered adding 8 grams of inulin daily to the diet of 48
young people increased the amount of calcium they absorbed
by around 20 percent. This also meant their bone mineral density (BMD) scores improved. A BMD test measures the amount
of good minerals in your bones and gives your doctor an idea of
your fracture risk.

But remember, you can't absorb enough calcium if you don't get
enough calcium. The recommended daily amount for men is
1,000 milligrams (mg) until age 71. After that, up your total to
1,200 mg. Women over 50 should aim for 1,200 mg, too.

Take the first step toward stronger bones. A nutrient-packed
breakfast that includes a cup of chicory coffee and calcium-
fortified cereal with milk can get you to your goal.

Inulin boosts weight loss. Inulin and a similar type of fiber
called oligofructose, help regulate ghrelin, also known as the
hunger hormone. Ghrelin's job is to increase your appetite. Cut
down the ghrelin, and you cut your chances of overeating. The
inulin and oligofructose in chicory lower ghrelin levels, so you
are not as hungry.

Here's proof. During one three-month study, people who took an oligofructose supplement every day lost a little over two pounds — and they reported feeling less hungry. Those who didn't get oligofructose? They gained almost a pound. Oops.

Inulin supports good digestion. Inulin is a prebiotic that passes through your digestive tract without being absorbed. As it travels through your system, it feeds your healthy microflora — the good bacteria living in your gut. So what's that mean for you? A reduced risk of colon cancer, less inflammation, and improved immune function.

Stronger bones, weight loss, and a healthy gut. A triple crown of benefits for a hale and hearty life.

Chicory root steadies your blood sugar

Are your blood sugar levels not exactly what the doctor ordered? Chicory root can give you a hand with that.

In a small Japanese study, researchers tested the A1c levels of people who drank chicory root extract every day for four weeks. The hemoglobin A1c — or HbA1c— number reflects the amount of glucose that's attached to molecules in your red blood cells. The thicker the coat of sugar on those cells, the higher your blood sugar, and the higher your A1c.

Half of those in this study drank a solution made from about 1/3 ounce of dried chicory root steeped in 1 1/2 cups of hot water. The other half were given a placebo mixture. Those who drank the chicory root extract improved their A1c three times more than the group who didn't drink chicory.

And there's more good news. The researchers also discovered that adiponectin — a protein that helps regulate your body's blood sugar levels — improved in the chicory group. Low levels of adiponectin are often found in people with insulin resistance.

Researchers believe chicory root extract could help delay — or even prevent — the early onset of diabetes.

Hidden inulin can cause digestive distress

Are you FODMAP-sensitive? If you suffer from Irritable Bowel Syndrome (IBS), you may already be familiar with the acronym FODMAP — Fermentable Oligosaccharides, Disaccharides, Monosaccharides, and Polyols. These are specific types of carbohydrates that trigger digestive discomfort in some people — like frequent diarrhea, bloating, and abdominal pain.

Sadly, FODMAP foods include some of your favorite healthy fruits and veggies like mushrooms, cauliflower, apples, pears — and, unfortunately — chicory root's fiber, inulin. It's classified as an oligosaccharide, the "O" in FODMAP.

If you're steering clear of FODMAPs, you'll want to avoid other inulin-containing foods like bananas, asparagus, onions, and Jerusalem artichokes, too.

Inulin has a neutral taste, so it's often used in place of sugar, fat, flour, or fiber in processed foods. It can be hiding in dairy products, breakfast cereals, breads, and other baked goods.

To keep inulin from sneaking into your diet, check nutrition labels carefully for inulin, chicory root, chicory root extract, or chicory root fiber.

Chilies

3 fabulous fat-burning foods

If you can stand the heat, get into the kitchen and chop up chili peppers. They not only add zing to your dishes, they burn calories, too. Here's how.

Chilies are chock-full of capsaicin, that powerful chemical that makes you cry for mercy from its spicy hot blow. It also curbs your appetite, making it a weight-loss wonder.

People who added red chili pepper to their meals felt satisfied and fuller for longer, discovered a research team in the Netherlands. A Purdue University study showed similar results.

"We found that consuming red pepper can help manage appetite and burn more calories after a meal," says Dr. Richard Mattes, a Purdue foods and nutrition professor, "especially for individuals who do not consume the spice regularly."

It's because capsaicin triggers a special protein that sends signals from your stomach to your brain, telling it that it's full. Not a bad way to kick-start your diet. Add these capsaicin-filled foods to your meals and watch the pounds melt away.

- Sriracha sauce. Sprinkle it on everything — really. Think eggs, popcorn, hummus, pretzels, almonds, tacos, and guacamole. Substitute it for ketchup. Add a few drops to vegetable juice. Savor the sizzle.

- Cayenne powder. Add bursts of flavor to your favorite soups, stews, and pasta dishes with cayenne powder. For a meal that tastes too sweet, add a dash of cayenne to tone it down.

- Chili peppers. Fall in love with roasted chili peppers. Toss small peppers onto a pan lined with foil. Cut the tops and bottoms off larger peppers and remove the insides. Slit in half and press flat. Don't remove the skins yet or you risk losing some of the flavor.

  Broil until charred on both sides. Place in a bowl and cover with plastic wrap for 20 minutes, allowing the peppers to steam. Remove the skins.

7 aches and pains you should never ignore

Ever feel pain in your chest after eating chili peppers? If you're reading this, then you know it was just heartburn — not a heart attack. But pain that persists in your chest needs medical attention pronto. In fact, you should never dismiss any of the following symptoms, because they could be a sign of something serious.

Symptom	What it could be
pain in chest, jaw, neck, shoulder, arm	heart attack
leg pain and swelling	deep-vein thrombosis
sudden severe headache	brain aneurysm
throbbing tooth	oral bacteria can increase risk of other diseases like stroke or cancer
sharp pain on your side	appendicitis, ovarian cyst
pins and needles	nerve damage
abdominal discomfort with gas or bloating	ovarian cancer

Hot peppers take a bite out of deadly diseases

Turn up the heat to defeat "the big three." People who ate fresh chili peppers almost every day slashed their risk of death from cancer, heart disease, and diabetes by 14 percent, found a study published in the *British Medical Journal.*

Even people who ate the hot stuff a couple times a week lowered their risk by 10 percent. It's all thanks to capsaicin, the substance that puts the "pep" in peppers.

If you fall into the group the study compared them to — those who eat chili peppers less than once a week — it's time to spice up your life.

Capsaicin puts the kibosh on cancer cells. What if you could take the compound in chilies that torches your taste buds and use it to crush cancer? You can. Experts say capsaicin suppresses stomach and colon tumors and can help wipe out melanoma.

A study published in *The Journal of Clinical Investigation* shows just how potent capsaicin is. Mice prone to deadly gut tumors lived a whopping 30 percent longer after eating capsaicin.

The scorching chemical works in the gut by helping to keep cells in the intestinal lining from multiplying too fast and turning into tumors. It protects the skin by blocking the growth and spread of melanoma cells and making them self-destruct.

Chilies boost heart health by improving blood flow. Past research suggests chili peppers lower blood pressure and block blood clots from forming. Now you can add high cholesterol to the list of heart problems the fiery food helps.

Chinese scientists recently discovered capsaicin breaks down cholesterol in your arteries, boosting blood flow to your heart and other organs.

"Our research has reinforced and expanded knowledge about how these substances in chilies work in improving heart health," says Dr. Zhen-Yu Chen, food and nutritional science professor at the Chinese University of Hong Kong. "We concluded that capsaicinoids were beneficial in improving a range of factors related to heart and blood vessel health."

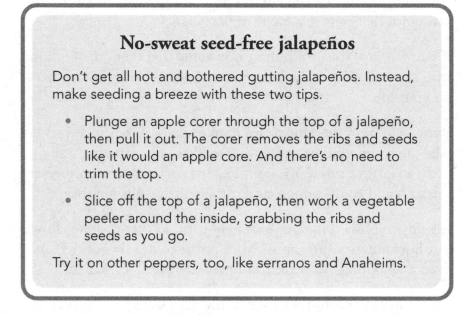

No-sweat seed-free jalapeños

Don't get all hot and bothered gutting jalapeños. Instead, make seeding a breeze with these two tips.

- Plunge an apple corer through the top of a jalapeño, then pull it out. The corer removes the ribs and seeds like it would an apple core. And there's no need to trim the top.

- Slice off the top of a jalapeño, then work a vegetable peeler around the inside, grabbing the ribs and seeds as you go.

Try it on other peppers, too, like serranos and Anaheims.

Fiery fare helps control blood sugar. Your skin, nerves, and joints have a pain receptor called TRPV1. When you regularly eat capsaicin or apply it to your skin, it overwhelms the pain receptors and often kills them, so you experience less pain. What does that have to do with diabetes?

Looks like blocking TRPV1 may also help you control your blood sugar by improving insulin response, say California researchers. Scientists know the TRPV1 receptors in nerve fibers around the pancreas prevent insulin from being released. Without insulin, sugar builds up in your bloodstream.

They studied aging mice that lacked the pain receptor and learned these animals could quickly remove sugar from their blood. They theorize that without TRPV1, the pancreas worked normally to keep blood sugar stable.

The mice also burned more calories without ramping up their exercise. That's great news since weight loss lowers diabetes risk.

"We think that blocking this pain receptor and pathway could be very, very useful," says Andrew Dillin, a professor of molecular and cell biology at the University of California. "Not only for relieving pain, but for improving life span and metabolic health, and in particular for treating diabetes and obesity in humans."

Go for the heat to cool chronic pain

Move over pain pills. Capsaicin delivers topical relief that's hard to beat.

When you apply capsaicin cream to your skin, it zaps substance P, a chemical that tells your brain, "Ouch, this hurts!" The less substance P you have, the less pain you feel, especially if you suffer from arthritis, shingles, diabetic nerve pain, backaches, or psoriasis.

Sounds like a miracle cure, but capsaicin creams take some getting used to. Some people find the initial sting hurts more than their chronic pain.

As long as you don't suffer serious side effects like blistering or swelling, stick with it by rubbing a thin layer of cream daily with cotton balls or latex gloves. Steer clear of your eyes, nose, mouth, and private parts. Go ahead and wash your hands afterwards.

For achy fingers, massage hands with cream, but don't wash right away. Give the medication at least 30 minutes to work before rinsing.

Daily application will desensitize your nerves, but it may take up to two months.

You could opt for over-the-counter capsaicin patches sold at your local drug store or online. These have .025 percent of capsaicin, just enough to soothe sore spots for up to eight hours.

Or talk to your doctor about prescription patches. One study found just one patch with a high concentration of capsaicin, 8 percent, calmed nerve pain for up to 12 weeks.

Crank up the flavor with spicy dried peppers

What can you do with dried chilies? Plenty. Drying chilies boosts their flavor, sweetness, and intensity, which adds an extra sizzle to all your dishes. And drying them is cheap and easy.

3 ways to dry chilies and savor the flavor. If you enjoy the heat from fresh hot peppers, you'll love the dry variety even more. Here are three easy ways to do it yourself.

- Super simple way — cook in the oven. Place chilies in a single layer on a baking sheet, and cook at 140 to 200 degrees for about eight hours. Rotate them throughout the day. For thick peppers, slice them open so the insides dry out faster.

- Super fun way — make a Mexican *ristra*. String your chilies with twine or fishing line threaded through a needle. Knot one end and push the needle through each pepper just below the stem. Hang in a hot, dry area for at least two weeks and up to six months.

- Super sunny way — dry them outdoors. Place peppers in a single layer on a plate or baking sheet outside in direct sunlight for several days. Make sure there's no rain in the forecast!

Take your dried peppers to a whole new level. Oh, the places peppers will go! With just a little imagination, you can score feisty flavors in just about anything. Here are a few ideas to get you started.

- Make your own fresh pepper flakes by coarsely grinding dried chilies in a blender.

- Finely grind them in a food processor or coffee grinder, and add to fresh rubs and marinades or soups and stews.

- Mix in a blender with olive oil, and drizzle over pasta, pizza, or stir-fries.

- Infuse small, dried peppers with vinegar to make a hot sauce for cooked greens.

- Make a paste by puréeing dried peppers with fresh water in a blender. Stir into homemade hummus, salad dressings, or over freshly grilled corn with a pat of butter.

Protect your peepers from potent peppers

If you've ever rubbed your eyes after chopping hot peppers, you've felt the burn. Not cool. Here's what to do if it happens again.

- Immediately wash your hands with dishwashing liquid to break down the peppers' oils. Or try rinsing them with vinegar.

- Flush out your eye with saline, eye drops, or plain water.

- If that doesn't cool the burn, dampen a clean cloth with milk and hold it over your eye for five minutes.

Better yet, practice an ounce of prevention. Wear latex gloves while slicing peppers, or soak fingertips in milk or yogurt when you're done chopping.

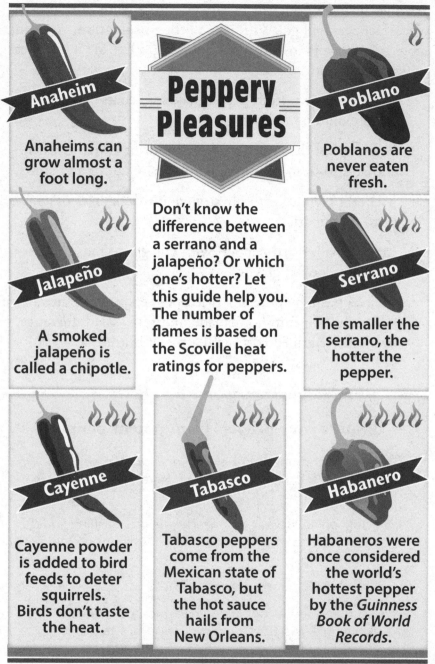

Peppery Pleasures

Don't know the difference between a serrano and a jalapeño? Or which one's hotter? Let this guide help you. The number of flames is based on the Scoville heat ratings for peppers.

Anaheim
Anaheims can grow almost a foot long.

Poblano
Poblanos are never eaten fresh.

Jalapeño
A smoked jalapeño is called a chipotle.

Serrano
The smaller the serrano, the hotter the pepper.

Cayenne
Cayenne powder is added to bird feeds to deter squirrels. Birds don't taste the heat.

Tabasco
Tabasco peppers come from the Mexican state of Tabasco, but the hot sauce hails from New Orleans.

Habanero
Habaneros were once considered the world's hottest pepper by the *Guinness Book of World Records*.

= mild   = medium   = hot   = scorching

Cinnamon

This bark can take a serious bite out of Alzheimer's

The smell of warm cinnamon wafting through the kitchen can only mean one thing — someone has been baking. And is there anything better than a fresh apple pie or a warm plate of cookies? For cinnamon lovers, here's news that could be the icing on the cake. Scientists think this fragrant spice could help ward off Alzheimer's Disease (AD).

The exact cause of AD remains unclear, but experts know the early warning signs — twisted, tangled fibers inside brain cells and sticky clumps of protein called plaque between brain cells. But cinnamon, a spice made from the inner bark of several types of the *Cinnamomum* tree, offers some powerful protection. All varieties contain a compound, cinnamaldehyde, that fights back against these dangerous knots.

Cinnamon improved the working memory of people over age 60 with prediabetes, shows a study published in the journal *Nutrition Research*. Ground cinnamon also prompted mice who were "poor learners" to have better recall by actually boosting levels of brain chemicals responsible for memories and decreasing other chemicals that interfere with brain function.

Researchers from University of California, Santa Barbara discovered cinnamaldehyde protects your brain from free radical damage called oxidative stress, and keeps proteins from massing together. Think of it a bit like sunblock, but for AD. Sunscreen prevents ultraviolet (UV) radiation from causing skin cancer.

Cinnamaldehyde helps prevent the dangerous brain changes connected to AD.

When you bake with cinnamon, you lose a bit of its spiciness, an indication some of the cinnamaldehyde has broken down. So to get the most benefit — and more flavor — sprinkle it straight into dishes and beverages, like your oatmeal or coffee.

Because these studies are still in their infancy, experts don't know how much cinnamon you need to work into your diet to get the maximum effect. Stay tuned for more information.

Trust your nose to save your spices

Have you ever been rooting through your pantry, only to find a jar of dried spices with a freshness label months old? Before you run to the store, make sure it's really time to replace it.

Dried spices get their flavors from the same oils that make them aromatic. But eventually, these oils evaporate away. So unlike milk or vegetables, dried spices don't actually spoil. They just lose color, flavor, and aroma over time. That means old spices won't give you food poisoning, but they could leave your dinner tasting pretty flat. Cook's tip — if they don't smell pungent, they won't be flavorful.

This evaporation process can take anywhere from months to years, depending on how you store your spices. Humid, warm, and bright places will speed up the evaporation, so it's best to keep them in a dark, cool spot.

Spice up your medicine cabinet to battle infections

Cinnamon is called an antimicrobial because natural compounds in it battle the bacteria behind a mixed bag of misery — everything from bad breath to food poisoning. In fact, traditional medicines around the world have used cinnamon for centuries to treat complaints like these. But it's in wound care that astonishing new discoveries are being made.

- Most recently, Japanese researchers isolated a specific polyphenol in true — or Ceylon — cinnamon called cinnamtannin B-1. This naturally occurring plant chemical did remarkable things when used to treat wounds in lab mice. It triggered certain stem cells to travel to the injury site much faster than normal, which led to a speedier healing time.

- One Malaysian study found a certain cinnamon extract from a local variety of the *Cinnamomum* tree was especially powerful against methicillin-resistant *Staphylococcus aureus* or MRSA, a particularly nasty bacterium unaffected by most antibiotics.

- American and Australian scientists joined forces to develop a new wound treatment packaged in microscopic capsules, combining cinnamaldehyde from cinnamon with peppermint oil. These work together to stimulate cells called fibroblasts, which are vital to tissue repair. There's hope this formula could be used as a topical antimicrobial and disinfectant.

Now, this doesn't mean you should keep cinnamon in your first aid kit. But soon you might be able to harness all of cinnamon's medicinal powers to stop infections and heal your cuts, bumps, and scrapes.

Hold your horses — true cinnamon won't blunt blood sugar

Cinnamon seems like a great tool to help you fight diabetes. After all, around two teaspoons of this spice can help you manage your blood sugar. But most grocery store cinnamon — probably Cassia or Chinese cinnamon — contains a potentially dangerous natural compound called coumarin. It's fine in small doses, but if you're taking cinnamon every day, it could be harmful, especially if you have liver problems.

You could switch to true cinnamon, also called Ceylon cinnamon, since this variety has very low levels of coumarin. But wait, human studies show that it has almost no effect on blood sugar.

What to do? Keep sprinkling Ceylon cinnamon on your morning oatmeal, since it is chock-full of healthy ingredients. Just don't rely on it to help treat your diabetes.

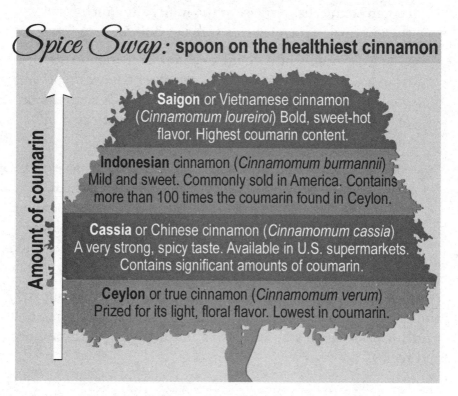

Spice Swap: **spoon on the healthiest cinnamon**

Amount of coumarin

Saigon or Vietnamese cinnamon (*Cinnamomum loureiroi*) Bold, sweet-hot flavor. Highest coumarin content.

Indonesian cinnamon (*Cinnamomum burmannii*) Mild and sweet. Commonly sold in America. Contains more than 100 times the coumarin found in Ceylon.

Cassia or Chinese cinnamon (*Cinnamomum cassia*) A very strong, spicy taste. Available in U.S. supermarkets. Contains significant amounts of coumarin.

Ceylon or true cinnamon (*Cinnamomum verum*) Prized for its light, floral flavor. Lowest in coumarin.

This flavor-filled spice could put the brakes on Parkinson's

Climbing Mount Everest seems like a less daunting task than taking on Parkinson's disease (PD). After all, this condition has no known cause or cure. So how do you even begin to protect yourself? Research published in the *Journal of Neuroimmune Pharmacology* reports the answer may lie in one of the world's oldest spices — cinnamon.

Even though experts don't know what causes Parkinson's, they know how it attacks your brain. It goes after neurons and chemical messengers, eventually leading to tremors, stiffness, balance problems, and walking issues.

In a mouse study, Rush University Medical Center researchers discovered both Cassia and Ceylon cinnamon have weapons that could help you fight back. They found ground cinnamon was metabolized into a compound called sodium benzoate, which protected neurons and held off the progression of Parkinson's.

The verdict is still out on how effective this treatment is for people, and how much cinnamon will help, but the outlook is promising. "Now we need to translate this finding to the clinic and test ground cinnamon in patients with PD," says lead researcher Kalipada Pahan, Ph.D. "If these results are replicated in PD patients, it would be a remarkable advance in the treatment of this devastating neurodegenerative disease."

Banish mold without burning your plants

Fuzzy, white mold growing on the soil of your potted plants is more than unsightly — it's dangerous. It introduces harmful allergens into your home, all while robbing your plants of their nutrients.

Some treatments will kill the mold, but they might kill your plants, too. Fortunately, the cinnamaldehyde in most commercial cinnamon has potent antimicrobial and fungicidal properties that can help you fight back against the mold without losing your favorite flowers.

- Scrape up all the mold you can see and throw it away.

- Add a fresh layer of potting soil to replace what you took out.

- Sprinkle the new soil with a layer of ground cinnamon to keep your plants mold-free.

Cocoa

Stay sharp with a sweet elixir

Over 60? Then you should be drinking cocoa every day. Those who did improved their memory and thinking in no time. Here's why.

Cocoa maintains a youthful brain. Italian researchers tested thinking, reasoning, and memory skills in men and women between the ages of 61 and 85. Then the scientists asked them to drink cocoa with varying amounts of flavanols every day for eight weeks. Flavanols are powerful compounds in plant-based foods that benefit your health.

Those who drank the cocoa with higher amounts of flavanols scored the best when they retook the tests at the end of the study. Experts aren't sure why, but they think it's because flavanols relax and widen blood vessels, boosting blood flow to your brain.

They also believe flavanols improve your body's insulin sensitivity, which helps keep your blood sugar stable. Glucose, or blood sugar, is your brain's main source of fuel. Keeping it in balance helps slow down brain aging.

Cocoa puts the brakes on Alzheimer's. This sweet elixir also battles the devastating effects of Alzheimer's disease on your brain. And once again, flavanols get the credit.

Flavanols prevent harmful substances like the protein beta-amyloid from building up in your brain, says a paper published in the *Journal of Alzheimer's Disease*.

For your mind to stay sharp, it needs to keep synapses snapping and communication flowing between nerve cells. Beta-amyloids form plaques that block the nerve cells and stop the process dead in its tracks.

The research with cocoa flavanols looks so promising, scientists want to explore using them to prevent and treat Alzheimer's in the future.

Bite-sized way to supercharge your workouts

If you had to choose between beetroot juice and dark chocolate for an exercise boost, which would you pick? Sounds like a trick question, but it's not.

"Beetroot juice is rich in nitrates, which are converted to nitric oxide in the body," explains Rishikesh Patel, a post-graduate student at Kingston University in London. "This dilates blood vessels and reduces oxygen consumption, allowing athletes to go further for longer."

The problem is, beetroot juice doesn't appeal to everyone. So a research team led by Patel asked a small group of amateur cyclists to trade one of their usual daily snacks for about 1 1/2 ounces of dark chocolate. They tested their performance after two weeks. Guess what happened?

Dark chocolate improved athletic performance just like the beet juice. The best part is, researchers say dark chocolate may supercharge any form of moderate exercise. Just make sure to count your calories.

Stay calm and eat dark chocolate

Feeling stressed? Reach for a piece of dark chocolate. It's the easy, no-drug solution to soothing frazzled nerves.

People who ate about 1 1/2 ounces of dark chocolate a day for two weeks had lower levels of the stress hormones cortisol and catecholamines, Swiss scientists discovered.

What's more, dark chocolate triggered the production of serotonin, your "feel-good" hormone. And get this — none of the people in the study experienced bad side effects like a rise in blood sugar. Sweet!

Experts say it has something to do with the wonderful way dark chocolate affects your gut's bacteria and your body's metabolism.

Not only did everyone in the study feel better, those who felt the highest anxiety levels at the beginning of the study benefitted the most.

Plus, you probably don't realize stress is the secret cause of excess belly fat, sleeplessness, and high blood pressure. Take a look at what the experts say.

- Anxiety leads to overeating and stress on your metabolism, which boosts belly fat.

- Stress is the No. 1 reason people can't fall asleep or stay asleep.

- Worry makes your body produce higher levels of stress hormones like epinephrine, which increases your heart rate and raises your blood pressure.

Makes you want to nibble a piece right now, doesn't it? If you want to mimic the Nestle-sponsored study, get dark chocolate with 74 percent cocoa solids. It's not hard to find — just read labels and look for the percentage of cocoa printed on the package.

And don't overdo it. Eating dark chocolate means adding fat and calories to your diet. Savor a small 3/4-ounce piece mid-morning and mid-afternoon.

Chop baking chocolate sans all the shavings

What's not to love about baking with chocolate? Nothing, except for the spray of shards when you slice into a bitter-sweet block. It's like taking a chain saw to a brick. Here's how to chop chocolate without making a mess.

Anchor your cutting board on a damp paper towel to keep it from slipping. For even less mess, place a rimmed baking sheet on the damp towel, and lay your cutting board inside it.

It also helps to slightly warm the chocolate. Microwave your chocolate bar in short spurts until the corners start to glisten.

Place the softened bar on the cutting board, and slice away with a serrated knife. It grabs the surface more easily than a straight blade and is perfect for finely chopped chocolate.

Enjoy having less cleanup and more chocolate for all your baking needs.

Cocoa makes the heart grow fonder

Chocolate and hearts go hand-in-hand, and not just on Valentine's Day. A little chocolate every day will keep your heart beating for years to come.

Flavanols get high-fives for fighting heart disease. That's what two separate studies proved when they tested cocoa drinks on healthy adults up to 80 years old. Participants drank beverages with or without cocoa flavanols twice a day for either two or four weeks.

At the end of both studies, those who drank the real cocoa showed one or more of the following:

- lower blood pressure

- better blood flow

- lower bad LDL cholesterol and higher good HDL cholesterol

- flexible blood vessels

- lower risk of heart disease

According to researcher Malte Kelm, cardiology professor at University Hospital Düsseldorf, cocoa can have long-term benefits for your heart.

"Our results indicate that dietary flavanol intake reduces the 10-year risk of being diagnosed with CVD (cardiovascular disease) by 22 percent and the 10-year risk of suffering a heart attack by 31 percent," he says.

Cocoa tops the charts for heart benefits. Based on previous studies, scientists know cocoa flavanols help people who are at high risk or who already have heart disease. These two studies focused on low-risk adults with no signs of heart problems. As you can see, the results show flavanols benefit healthy adults, too.

So no matter what group you fall into — healthy, at-risk, or diagnosed with heart disease — you can drink cocoa to your heart's content. But before you raid the pantry for your favorite hot cocoa mix, listen up. It's the natural, unsweetened powder that's good for you, not the sugary stuff you top with marshmallows and whipped cream on cold, wintry nights.

Unsweetened cocoa powder contains the highest number of flavanols and won't add inches to your waist. One tablespoon has only 12 calories. Other chocolate products have fewer flavanols because of the way they're processed.

Ranked from highest to lowest in flavanols are cocoa powder, baking chocolate, dark chocolate or baking chips, milk chocolate, and chocolate syrup. Notice the pattern? The sweeter the chocolate, the fewer nutrients it contains.

More cocoa? Yes, please! Finding ways to add unsweetened cocoa to your diet is the best way to boost your flavanol intake. These ideas will get you started.

- Mix frozen banana slices and cocoa powder in a blender until smooth for a creamy treat.

- Make granola bars with rolled oats, your favorite nut butter, a little honey or agave syrup, chopped nuts or seeds, and a dusting of cocoa powder.

- Sprinkle over popcorn while you catch up on your favorite flicks.

- Add a tablespoon to a pot of beef stew or chili.

- Toss cocoa powder in with your homemade barbecue sauce, and baste it on grilled chicken.

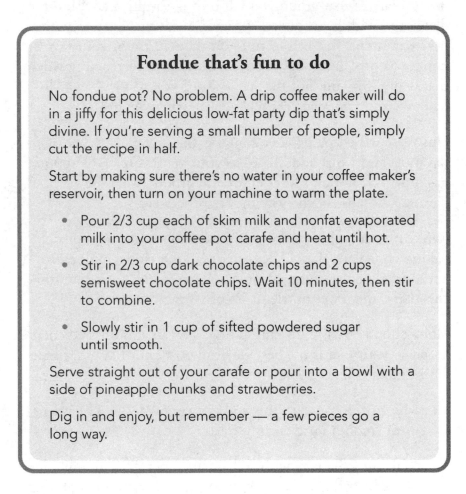

Fondue that's fun to do

No fondue pot? No problem. A drip coffee maker will do in a jiffy for this delicious low-fat party dip that's simply divine. If you're serving a small number of people, simply cut the recipe in half.

Start by making sure there's no water in your coffee maker's reservoir, then turn on your machine to warm the plate.

- Pour 2/3 cup each of skim milk and nonfat evaporated milk into your coffee pot carafe and heat until hot.

- Stir in 2/3 cup dark chocolate chips and 2 cups semisweet chocolate chips. Wait 10 minutes, then stir to combine.

- Slowly stir in 1 cup of sifted powdered sugar until smooth.

Serve straight out of your carafe or pour into a bowl with a side of pineapple chunks and strawberries.

Dig in and enjoy, but remember — a few pieces go a long way.

From beans to bonbons: the story behind this healthy passion

Before it becomes a melt-in-your-mouth bar or a bonbon, chocolate starts out as a bean from the cacao plant. Once the beans are dried and roasted, the inner nibs are removed and ground into a liquor made of 55 percent cocoa butter. This liquor is processed into your favorite chocolates and cocoa powder.

But with dozens of varieties to choose from, how do you know what you're getting? Use this guide to help you.

Sweet guide to all things chocolate

	Milk chocolate	Smooth taste, but loaded with milk fat and cocoa butter.
	Dark chocolate	Must have at least 35 percent cacao, but check labels for higher amounts. The higher the percentage, the more flavanols you get.
	White chocolate	Tastes creamy, but made with cocoa butter, milk, and sugar, and void of nutrients.
	Semi-sweet chocolate	Versatile and great for baking (and snacking!)
	Bittersweet chocolate	Made mostly of chocolate liquor, so it's high in flavanols.
	Mexican chocolate	Dark, loaded with flavanols, and flavored with almonds, vanilla, and cinnamon. Makes the best hot cocoa ever!
Cocoa powder	Natural	High in flavanols, low in fat and sugar, strong bitter taste.
	Dutch	Also known as "alkalized" cocoa, it's low in flavanols due to the way it's processed.
	Lavado	Contains the most flavanols, but hard to find and pricey.

Coffee

Power up your brain with a cup o' joe

"I never drink coffee at lunch. I find it keeps me awake for the afternoon." Ronald Reagan understood the power of caffeine. A natural stimulant, it's found in over 60 plants, including the kola nut, tea leaf, cacao pod, and — perhaps the world's favorite source — coffee beans. Humorously nicknamed "the other vitamin C" for its famous energy kick, caffeine can do much more than just jolt you awake in the morning.

Boost your brain power. Researchers think caffeine works in your brain like this.

Ordinarily, a natural chemical in your body called adenosine links up with areas on cells called adenosine receptors, and triggers a reaction that causes you to slow down and feel sleepy.

But when you drink coffee, the caffeine molecules that enter your bloodstream are so similar to adenosine, they can take their place on these receptors. The caffeine molecules don't trigger the same reaction, however, so your body doesn't get the message to fall asleep.

You continue to feel energetic and alert. Thanks, caffeine.

Lower your risk for dementia. In a study of nearly 6,500 women over age 65, those who drank the equivalent of two or three 8-ounce cups of regular coffee every day reduced their risk of developing dementia by a whopping 36 percent compared to the women who drank less.

So don't let your brain deteriorate when you can so easily power it up. Go ahead. Enjoy another delicious cup. As far as your brain's concerned, it's good to the last drop.

Goats, monks, and prayers: how the brew began

It all started over 1,000 years ago with dancing goats on a hillside far, far away. Legend says Ethiopian goatherd Kaldi watched in amazement as his flock gleefully frolicked about after they nibbled on red berries from a coffee shrub. Not wanting to miss out on the fun, Kaldi stuffed some berries in his own mouth, too.

Soon a monk wandered by, observed the energetic cavorting of Kaldi and his goat friends, and promptly carried some of the coffee berries back to his drowsy brothers at the monastery. That evening at vespers, the monks were delighted to discover the berries helped them stay awake during even the longest prayers. History has credited these caffeinated monks with being the first to boil the berries, producing the brew now served 'round the world.

Beneficial bean de-'livers' surprising protection

What weighs a little more than 3 pounds, is shaped like a flat football, and has a to-do list of more than 300 tasks that keep your body humming along? Your liver, of course. This second largest organ in your body — only your skin is larger — turns the food you eat into energy and nutrients. Plus it filters out harmful substances. Want to give this unglamorous organ the TLC it deserves? Just have another cup of coffee.

Fat overload leads to liver damage. Your liver naturally contains some fat. That's normal. But when fat is more than 5 to 10 percent of your liver's total weight, you're diagnosed with a fatty liver.

Nonalcoholic fatty liver disease (NAFLD), the leading type of chronic liver disease in the U.S., affects up to one in four adults. And it's serious. This disease can lead to cirrhosis, liver cancer, and even liver failure.

The condition is most common in people who are overweight or obese, but there are other risk factors, too, like diabetes, high cholesterol, and high triglycerides. Surprisingly, poor eating habits, including rapid weight loss, can also lead to NAFLD.

Symptoms of the illness can be vague, if you have any at all. However, you may experience fatigue, nausea, abdominal pain, itching, and confusion. Your doctor may suspect the disease if your blood tests show high levels of certain enzymes. And he may order an ultrasound to confirm his diagnosis.

Bet you didn't know your steaming mug is packed with chlorogenic acid (CGA), a powerful antioxidant that protects you from diabetes, cancer, and even dementia. But be sure to choose the right roast. Research shows lightly roasted beans can contain up to 25 times more CGA than the average dark roast.

Coffee brews up liver benefits. In a study of 155 people with NAFLD, researchers found those who drank two or more cups of coffee daily had less liver stiffness — and that means a lower risk of liver disease. Caffeine may be the hero that keeps your liver healthy by reducing inflammation. But more research is needed before scientists will know for sure which of the thousands of coffee compounds — like chlorogenic acid (CGA), for example — should get the credit.

So far there's no cure for NAFLD. But if you stick to a healthy diet — including a couple cups of coffee — and exercise regularly, you may be able to reverse the disease in its early stages. Even better? With the right diet and lifestyle changes, you might be able to avoid NAFLD altogether.

A leaner creamer: mix up a lip-smacking alternative

Holy latte, Batman. That sweet, velvety creamer you just added to your coffee probably contains artificial flavors, thickeners, preservatives, sodium, saturated fat, and — oh yes — high fructose corn syrup. That last ingredient is, according to a study conducted by Duke University Medical Center, especially bad news for your liver.

"We found that increased consumption of high fructose corn syrup was associated with scarring in the liver, or fibrosis, among patients with nonalcoholic fatty liver disease (NAFLD)," says Manal Abdelmalek, associate professor of medicine.

Satisfy your craving — and keep your liver healthy — with this easy, make-at-home creamer recipe. In a lidded jar, combine:

- 1/2 cup regular half-and-half

- 1/4 cup unsweetened almond milk

- 1 tablespoon pure maple syrup

- 2 teaspoons vanilla extract

Adjust flavorings to taste. Shake creamer until well-blended. Store in your fridge for up to one week.

A 3-tablespoon serving adds about 60 calories to your cup. Not too bad, when you consider one well-known creamer stirs in 105 calories for the same serving size.

Your morning brew boosts good gut bacteria

Coffee companies ply their wares with slogans like, "Better beans. Better coffee." But now they can add the claim, "Better gut," to coffee's fame. Researchers have found your favorite morning blend is good medicine for the healthy bacteria in your intestines.

Your gut contains trillions of bacteria that impact not just your digestion, but how your body fights off disease as well. Called your microbiome, it's been linked to how you feel, how you think, and even how you age. Experts believe the greater the variety of bacteria in your microbiome, the healthier you are. You can help your gut make a change for the better by simply tweaking your diet.

One group of researchers looked at more than 1,100 people in the Netherlands and another examined 5,000 volunteers in Belgium. Their task? To find out how diet impacts the bacteria living in your microbiome.

These experts concluded what you eat and drink can change your bacteria for better or for worse. To increase your good gut bacteria, researchers recommend a diet rich in blueberries and other fruits, vegetables like beans, yogurt with live cultures, but-termilk, and — of course, coffee.

Amazingly, it could be java's soluble fiber that stirs up the helpful bacteria in your microbiome. Two friendly bacteria groups — Bacteroides and Prevotella — showed a 60-percent boost during the 24 hours they were exposed to coffee's fiber.

But be careful what you add to make your healthy brew tastier. Whole milk, artificial sweeteners, and processed foods like some coffee creamers squelch the good guys in your gut.

So go ahead and treat your microbiome to another cup of coffee. It triggers a gut reaction just brimming with great benefits.

This spice is right for a gentler java

Does your coffee spark stomach discomfort? There's no need to ditch your daily cup. Instead, savor the delicious flavor of Turkish coffee blended with cardamom — India's "Queen of Spices" — and nip those tummy troubles in the bud.

Known for its delicious aroma and breath-freshening qualities, time-honored cardamom has been used for centuries to treat stomach ailments. But modern researchers have uncovered another of ancient cardamom's spicy secrets. Turns out 3 grams of powdered cardamom a day — that's about 1 1/2 teaspoons — could significantly lower your blood pressure.

It's easy to add a little cardamom to your morning mug. For an eight-cup pot, just add 1 tablespoon of ground cardamom to 8 tablespoons of finely ground coffee. Brew as usual and enjoy a true Turkish delight.

Colon cancer: health perks by the cup

Experts estimate about 135,000 people will be diagnosed with colorectal cancer this year, and — tragically — more than 50,000 people will die. Coffee is by no means a cure for this frightening disease, but it is a weapon you can add to your anti-cancer arsenal.

Drink more than 2 1/2 cups of coffee every day, and you'll cut your chances of developing colorectal cancer by 54 percent. How? Coffee contains compounds that slow the growth of cancer cells, help your body quickly rid itself of cancer-causing substances, and defend against damaging free radicals.

8 kitchen scraps your plants will love to eat

Waste not, want not. This well-known proverb dates all the way back to the year 1576 when it began as the tongue-tripping, "Willful waste makes woeful want." Although the words have changed with the times, what was true almost 500 years ago, still holds true today — especially for your garden.

You may be tempted to toss out these eight kitchen scraps, but don't. The leftover nutrients hiding in these throwaways make first-rate fodder for hungry plants.

- Coffee grounds. Rich in nitrogen that enhances the soil, your daily grind can turn into a pick-me-up for your plants that also improves soil texture and drainage. Sprinkle a layer of used grounds no more than half an inch thick on your garden, work gently into the soil, and watch your plants perk right up. Camellias and azaleas will especially love the acid boost, but stay away from asparagus ferns and geraniums. Coffee's not their cup of tea. You may find used coffee grounds also repel pests like snails, slugs, squirrels, and even rabbits.

- Cooking water. Just finished boiling eggs, pasta, potatoes, or spinach? Don't pour that water down the drain. After it cools, treat your garden to a good long drink. Healthful nutrients — like starch, iron, calcium, and potassium — are left behind in the water. Just don't use water that has salt added. It could damage your plants.

- Banana peels. Are aphids a problem for your roses? Not if you have banana peels. Just cut them into small pieces — no more than 1/2 inch by 1/2 inch — and bury them around your rose bushes. Make sure they are well below the surface so raccoons and other snack-hungry critters won't come nosing around your garden, but don't disturb any roots. An added bonus. You love bananas for their potassium, and your roses will, too.

- Whole-grain cereal and bread crusts. To make your soil richer, bury these scraps in the ground near your plants or in the rows of your garden. Whole grains make a tasty treat for garden-friendly earthworms, but they keep harmful bugs at bay.

- Crushed shells. This long-lasting mulch adds calcium and other nutrients to your flower bed, vegetable garden, or flower pots. You can buy pre-crushed seashells at your local garden supplier. But if that gets too pricey, save the remains from your seafood dinner or ask for free shells at your favorite seafood restaurant, and crush them yourself.

Start by thoroughly washing and boiling the shells to remove excess salt. Next, cover large whole shells — like mussels, crabs, and oysters — with a cloth, and hammer them into smaller pieces. Since shells decay slowly, a two-inch layer of this mulch could last up to two years.

- Sour milk. Here's another rich source of calcium for your plants. Dilute sour milk with water and pour it at the base of your rosebushes or tomato plants. An extra benefit? The smell of sour milk chases away nibbling deer.

- Tea leaves. As a treat for acid-loving plants like rosebushes, rhododendrons, azaleas, blueberries, or ferns, surround each with a circle of tea leaves. Not only will they keep slugs away, but since they contain nutrients and tannic acid, they will boost your soil quality and help your plants grow stronger roots. You can also steep used tea bags and pour the cooled liquid around the base of these plants.

- Citrus peels. Lemon and orange peels juice up your plants by adding nitrogen, calcium, magnesium, and sulfur to the soil. Just let the peels dry, grind them up, and mix them into your garden. A frugal way to sweeten your plot.

Coffee flour — a nutritious break from your usual grind

There's coffee-flavored candy, ice cream, and yogurt. Or how about some coffee jelly for your morning toast? These are just a few of the treats coffee producers have cooked up to tempt fans of the bean.

But coffee flour? Tried that one yet? If not, you may want to give it a shot.

A bean with a mission. The morning mug you look forward to every day is brewed from seeds harvested from coffee cherries, the bright red fruit of the coffee plant. Once the beans have been removed, lots of plant pulp is left behind — and it usually ends up in rivers and streams, or it's left in giant heaps to rot. Not good for the environment. Or the local economy.

Enter today's scientists. They figured out how to use these plant leftovers in a way that cleans up the environment, creates jobs for coffee-growing communities, and provides the world with a delicious new food to enjoy.

Coffee flour is brimming with nutrition. According to the website *coffeeflour.com*, you'll get more fiber in their product than in an equal amount of whole-grain wheat flour. It's also a great source of iron and potassium. Plus it's gluten-free.

But beware. It's not completely caffeine-free. Coffee flour contains about the same amount of caffeine as dark chocolate. Or think of it this way — one tablespoon has roughly the caffeine content of 1/3 cup of black coffee.

Get cooking! You can use coffee flour in breads, cookies, and even homemade pastas. Since it's made from the coffee cherries, not the bean, coffee flour adds floral, citrusy notes to your dishes instead of the dark, robust flavors you might expect.

But don't do an even exchange of regular all-purpose flour for coffee flour. To get started, chefs in-the-know recommend replacing 10 to 15 percent of your all-purpose flour. You can adjust amounts from there.

Here are a few more important kitchen tips:

- Be sure to sift the flours together rather than adding them separately so the liquids will be absorbed evenly.

- You'll need to increase your liquid ingredients by 10 to 25 percent, too, because of all the fiber packed into coffee flour.

- Don't shorten baking times just because your cookies or muffins look overdone in the oven. That's the coffee flour's rich color coming through. Trust the timing given in your recipe.

> Not much of a baker, but still want to put coffee flour to the test? Switch out cocoa powder for coffee flour in your morning smoothie. Just a tablespoon or two will do the trick. Blend thoroughly and enjoy.

Coffee flour is a little pricey. A 1-pound bag will run you $8.99 at *nuts.com*, and an even smaller amount — a 1/2-pound bag — will cost you about that much on *amazon.com*. But as you can see, a little will go a long way.

Maybe you'd like to give the taste a try before you buy? Check out the special selection of baked goods made with coffee flour at your local Sprouts Farmers Market.

EGCG

It's green tea time! Steep to new levels of cancer protection

When you take the road to better health, green tea deserves a green light. It's the super healer that fights heart disease, promotes weight loss, battles cancer, and acts as an antioxidant to boost your immune system.

That's a lot of healing going on. Yet, the secret power in this popular and healthy beverage is one tiny, naturally occurring plant compound with a name tongue-twisting enough to leave you longing for Peter and his peck of pickled peppers — epigallocatechin-3-gallate. Don't worry about pronouncing it. Call it EGCG and just know it's the most active and studied substance in green tea.

EGCG signals good news against oral cancer. Roughly one person per hour, 24 hours a day will die from cancer of the lips, tongue, cheeks, sinuses, or throat. But Penn State researchers found evidence that EGCG could be a magic bullet against oral cancers like these.

They think it works by targeting a special protein called sirtuin 3 or SIRT3. When EGCG interacts with SIRT3 in cancer cells, the cells die. But when it hooks up with SIRT3 in normal cells, it makes them stronger and better able to protect themselves.

And here's the coolest news of all. "The idea that EGCG might selectively affect the activity of sirtuin 3 in cancer cells to turn it off — and in normal cells to turn it on — is probably applicable in multiple kinds of cancers," says Joshua Lambert, associate professor of food science at Penn State. That means this same process could work against other cancers.

Here's how to save your own skin. A lab study out of the University of Alabama proves the theory true. In this case, EGCG slayed skin cancer cells while leaving the rest of the skin cells alone, by specifically blocking a cancer-promoting protein called beta-catenin. It also tackled the chronic inflammation that can trigger the production of skin cancer cells.

> Most studies of EGCG don't use tea. Scientists run tests using extracts or supplements because they usually work in laboratories or on animals.

These are just two cancers EGCG fights. But the research doesn't end there. A review of several studies published in the medical journal *Nutrition* shows this powerful polyphenol also attacks lung cancer, gastric cancer, colon cancer, breast cancer, and prostate cancer.

While green tea is the richest source of EGCG, you can also find it in smaller amounts in other teas.

Let your cup runneth over with EGCG

Just a few basics will help you get the most bang for your buck. The following table lists teas in order from highest to lowest EGCG content.

Green tea, loose leaf	Leaves are steamed soon after they're picked which preserves EGCG and other flavanols.
White tea	Named for the fuzzy white "needles" on the unopened buds of the tea bush used to make this deliciously mild drink.

Oolong tea	Leaves are "bruised" to help release their antioxidants.
Green tea, decaffeinated	Still can contain up to 12 milligrams of caffeine per cup.
Green tea, flavored	Available in a variety of fruity flavors from açai to wild berry.
Black tea	Leaves are fermented before drying, so they lose a lot of EGCG.
Black tea, flavored	Peach, candy apple, cranberry, passionfruit, and pomegranate — just a few fruit-flavored teas available.
Green tea, ready-to-drink	Careful. Bottled green teas can be loaded with sugar. Read labels carefully.
Black tea, instant powder	Cheap and convenient, but contains almost no EGCG.

Tonic in a teapot — look good, feel good

One of the oldest and most popular beverages in the world can make you look and feel like a million bucks. Know what it is? You guessed it — green tea, the mild-flavored drink with health benefits galore.

Whittle off weight and burn belly fat. Go ahead. Grab your skinny jeans. You're going to want to show this off. Experts say EGCG lowers the amount of fat your body absorbs and helps you eliminate it. Plus, the combo of EGCG and caffeine in green tea burns calories and breaks down belly fat. Need proof?

• When reviewing more than 26 trials from all over the world, experts discovered people who were normal weight or overweight shed pounds and inches by regularly drinking green tea or taking green tea extracts with caffeine.

- In a Chinese study of 182 moderately overweight people, researchers found those who drank the equivalent of six to 10 cups of green tea every day for three months not only lost weight, but also trimmed their middles.

Renew your veins and arteries naturally. Multiple studies out of Japan prove drinking several cups of green tea daily can lower your chances of stroke and dying from heart disease.

Scientists say catechins in green tea like EGCG block your body from absorbing cholesterol. Not only that, losing weight and belly fat helps out your heart, too.

Adrienne wants the benefits of EGCG without sitting down for tea time. Her solution? Green tea smoothies. It's easy. Make a pot of green tea and let it cool. The next time you whip up a smoothie, use the tea to replace your juice, water, milk, or other liquid.

Say bye-bye to dangerous BP. Question: What do you get when you lose weight AND lower your cholesterol? Answer: Lower blood pressure. They go hand-in-hand. So just by accomplishing the first two, green tea helps you achieve the second. But in addition, EGCG performs its own unique magic on your blood pressure by keeping the inner lining of your blood vessels healthy and your heart's main chamber from thickening.

Green tea yields sweet pain relief

A warm cup of green tea soothes more than your soul. It calms achy joints, too. All thanks to the natural way EGCG keeps pain at bay.

Experts say this catechin works on multiple fronts as it battles arthritis. For one, it's an anti-inflammatory that targets those swollen spots, like your knees, hips, and shoulders. It's also "chon-droprotective" — a scientific way of saying it keeps the spaces between your joints from narrowing. And that means you're less likely to have bones rubbing painfully against other bones.

Scientists have gained their insights from animal studies like these.

- Osteoarthritis (OA). EGCG reduced pain, protected joints from cartilage breakdown, and slowed the progression of osteoarthritis, according to an article published in the journal *Arthritis Research & Therapy*. What's more, EGCG-treated mice had fewer substances in their bodies that promote inflammation.

- Rheumatoid arthritis (RA). EGCG blocked the destructive work of a protein called TAK1, discovered scientists out of Washington State University. This protein triggers a process that damages joints and tissue.

What do these two studies mean for you? Researchers hope to use EGCG as a healthier treatment for arthritis in the future.

"Existing drugs for rheumatoid arthritis are expensive," says Salah-uddin Ahmed, the lead Washington State researcher, "and sometimes unsuitable for long-term use." The same could be said of OA drugs.

7 tips to get the most out of your green tea

Want to brew the perfect cup? Follow these tips to maximize flavor and health benefits.

- Store green tea leaves in a sealed container in a dark, cool place.

- Throw out any you've had hanging around for over six months. They may have lost close to 30 percent of their EGCG. Fresh is best.

- Get more EGCG by using high-quality, loose-leaf tea instead of tea bags.

- Don't pour boiling water over green tea. You could burn the leaves. In fact, the Tea Association of the U.S.A. says after your water comes to a boil, remove it from the heat and allow to sit for 10 minutes. Then pour over your leaves.

- Steep green tea for about four minutes to get the most EGCG.

- If you do use a tea bag, stop squashing it against the inside of your cup with a spoon. This releases bitter-tasting tannins.

- Add a little zing to your tea with lemon, orange, lime, or grapefruit juice. Citrus juices help your body absorb more EGCG.

Smart brew boosts brain cells to a 'T'

You're never too old to learn something new. But just in case you need a little help with that — green tea to the rescue! It's an age-old remedy that promotes a youthful brain.

For years, research has shown green tea benefits your memory. But recent studies have given scientists a better idea of how it works.

One Chinese study, for instance, looked at how EGCG affects brain cells. "We focused our research on the hippocampus, the part of the brain which processes information from short-term to long-term memory," says Professor Yun Bai from the Third

Military Medical University. He and his team discovered this super antioxidant supercharges the formation of important cells.

Next, they tested their discovery on mice to see if the increase in cells helped them remember where to find hidden objects in a maze. The mice who received EGCG found the objects quicker than the mice who didn't get EGCG.

"This helps us to understand the potential for EGCG, and green tea which contains it, to help combat degenerative diseases and memory loss," says Bai.

Savor a cupful of heart health

What would happen if a city's main highway blew up? Bedlam, that's what.

Much like a city, your body has its own super highway, the aorta, a major artery supplying blood to your abdomen, pelvis, and legs. Doctors aren't sure what causes it to swell and stretch, a condition called an abdominal aortic aneurysm (AAA), but it's most often seen in men over 60 who smoke, have high blood pressure, or a family history of this condition.

Most troubling about AAAs is that they are difficult to detect, and, without treatment, the artery can rupture, leaving you with a scary 50 percent chance of survival.

Green tea can change all that. "The type of polyphenol found in green tea has recently been shown to regenerate elastin, an essential protein that gives the artery its stretchy, yet sturdy, texture," explains Shuji Setozaki of Kyoto University Graduate School of Medicine in Japan. After a lab study, researchers believe green tea could be a new preventive strategy for AAAs. Their focus in future studies will be to determine the best dose.

Say yes to tea and no to sugar spikes

Green tea and bagels may sound like a perfectly perfect breakfast combo to you. And they are a yummy way to start your day. But they go hand-in-hand for another reason besides taste. The EGCG in that cup of green tea can level out your blood sugar when you drink it with a high-carbohydrate item, like a bagel.

Normally, you eat something full of carbs and your digestive system breaks most of it down into sugar, which enters your bloodstream. This signals your pancreas to produce insulin, which helps your cells absorb the blood sugar for energy. The levels of sugar in your blood fall and your pancreas stops making insulin.

When this process, called carbohydrate metabolism, fails, insulin runs amok in your body and you're on the road to diabetes. That's why controlling spikes in blood sugar after eating carbohydrates is so important.

Penn State researchers fed mice cornstarch, a substance that raises blood sugar levels, plus a dose of EGCG equal to the amount in about 1 1/2 cups of green tea. Then they compared glucose levels to mice fed only cornstarch.

"The spike in blood glucose level is about 50 percent lower than the increase in the blood glucose level of mice that were not fed EGCG," says Joshua Lambert, a Penn State assistant professor of food science.

Scientists think it's because EGCG restricts the activity of alpha-amylase, an enzyme in your saliva and pancreas that turns starch into sugar.

"If what you are eating with your tea has starch in it," Lambert says, "then you might see that beneficial effect."

Essential oils

Massage: the healing power of touch

How would you feel if someone gave you frankincense and myrrh for your birthday? A bit of a letdown, right? Maybe not. These two gifts aren't just a symbol of royalty. People have used them to fight inflammation and pain for centuries. And they're not the only plant products with benefits fit for a king.

Walk through a rose garden or pine forest, and take a deep breath. You are smelling essential oils. To bottle them into the concentrated liquids found online or in stores, you first have to extract the oils from the leaves, stems, flowers, bark, or roots of a plant.

But make no mistake — essential oils are more than aromas. Often referred to as the life force of plants, some have the ability to heal, soothe, and even disinfect.

If you have aches and pains, try a soothing massage with frankincense, myrrh, and other essential oils — a gift that keeps on giving.

Drug-free power over pain. Why pair the power of plants with the benefits of massage? Essential oil molecules are tiny enough to absorb into your skin. They make their way to your bloodstream, where they go to work throughout your body.

That's not the only reason essential oil massages are a crowd favorite, though. They also help relax your muscles and soothe nerve endings. And don't forget how special you feel when you're pampered.

Eight oh-so-essential oils to bring you relief. Not just any essential oil will do, however. Some relieve pain and fight inflammation better than others. These are the most popular:

- black pepper
- eucalyptus
- ginger
- myrrh

- chamomile
- frankincense
- lavender
- rosemary

An essential rule for a safe massage. Rubbing a highly concentrated liquid on your skin probably makes you nervous, and for good reason. The effect of essential oils can be 100 times more potent than the original plants. No surprise, putting them directly on your skin could cause irritation or allergic reactions.

The solution is simple — carrier oils. Combined with essential oils, these protect your skin while helping you absorb the beneficial oils easily.

Common carrier oils include avocado, canola, coconut, grapeseed, jojoba, olive, sweet almond, and walnut oils as well as cocoa butter.

A generally safe rule is to use a 2 percent essential oil dilution on your skin. Don't worry, you don't have to do math. Simply add 12 drops of essential oil to each fluid ounce of carrier oil.

6 easy ways to get rid of back pain

You're no stranger to pain. From the twinge of a pulled muscle to the constant ache of a sore back, you've spent more than your fair share of time suffering. A nice massage with soothing essential oils could be your remedy of choice. But if you need more easy solutions you can do yourself, try one of these other five ways to send pain packing.

Put it on ice. If you just hurt your back, grab an ice pack or bag of frozen vegetables. Apply for 10 to 20 minutes every two hours for the first 48 hours to relieve pain and swelling.

Turn up the heat. After an injury, it's best to wait 48 hours before going for the heating pad or a hot bath. On the other hand, heat is great any time for relaxing muscles if you have a persistent backache.

Position your pillow properly. The way you sleep can make aches and pains worse, but the right pillow position could really change the game.

- For a backache, side sleepers should place a pillow between their bent knees to support the spine. If you sleep on your back, place the pillow under your knees.

- If you have pain that's cramping your upper back, shoulders, and neck, make sure your pillow is soft enough to conform to the curve of your neck. And avoid pillows that are too high or too stiff.

Did you know your pillow can also help you fight other causes of nighttime discomfort? To control heartburn, use a wedge-shaped pillow to prop up your head and torso at least six inches. If you suffer from leg cramps, use an extra pillow to elevate your legs.

Plank it out. A weak core puts your back in the injury danger zone. Do this exercise every day to strengthen your abdominal muscles and protect your back.

Important note — while the plank can minimize low back pain for many people, if you've suffered an injury, talk to your doctor or physical therapist before trying it.

- Get down on the floor, on your toes in the push-up position, with your hands shoulder-width apart.

- Keep your arms straight and your body in one long line.

- Contract all your muscles and hold for about 20 to 30 seconds.

- Rest and repeat.

If your back pain comes from scoliosis, a sideways curving of the spine, this classic side plank can help.

- Lie on your left side with your legs extended.

- Push up and straighten your left arm so you are supported by your left hand.

- Extend your right arm straight up, using a wall for support if needed.

- Raise your hips so your body is in a straight line from shoulders to ankles.

- Contract your stomach and leg muscles.

- Hold the position as long as possible, working up to 90 seconds.

- Repeat on your right side.

Is this classic side plank too difficult? Try a
modified version where you rest on one
elbow and keep your legs and hips on the
floor, lifting only your upper body.
Planking is easier than sit-ups,
and as a bonus, it can
help you flatten a
bulging belly.

Explore aquatics. Water helps support your weight, putting
less strain on your joints while offering gentle resistance. This
makes water workouts, also called hydrotherapy, great for people
with bone loss, joint pain, and muscle strains. Again, ask your
doctor what activities are safe for your type of back pain.

Cent-sational scents: how to get your money's worth

Top-notch essential oils can be hard to spot. Avoid the
scavenger hunt, and follow these smart buying tips.

- Look beyond the label. Don't be fooled into thinking
  terms like "therapeutic grade" or "certified" mean
  the product is golden. These claims are not regulated, so they don't mean much.

- Research the company. You want 100 percent pure
  essential oils that have been distilled properly. How
  can you tell? A reputable seller should know where the
  oils come from, how they are made, if they contain
  added ingredients, and if they are tested for quality.

- Compare price tags. You don't have to buy the most
  expensive oils, but you should be wary of amazing bargains. If the price is too low, it may not be the real deal.

The nose knows — aromatherapy for peace of mind

Stressed? Then stop and smell the roses. Literally. That sweet scent may help you relax and feel better say researchers. And that's what aromatherapy is all about, the use of plant oils to heal your body or change your mood.

Think of it this way. Your nose is always on standby. Any time the smell receptors in your sniffer get a whiff of something, they snap into action, sending signals to your brain — specifically the areas that store emotions and memories. That's how scientists think essential oils influence your physical and emotional health.

Waft away worry with calming aromas. Lavender, chamomile, sweet marjoram, bergamot, and sandalwood are essential oils that tell your nervous system to calm down. In fact, when nurses delivered aromatherapy as part of patient care during over 10,000 hospital visits, they found lavender and sweet marjoram were especially helpful in relieving anxiety. Who knew tranquility could be just a sniff away?

Doze off to sleepy-time smells. Better sleep leads to longer life. But for some, winding down at the end of the day takes effort. Luckily, aromatherapy, combined with good sleep habits, can improve the quality of your slumber, says a study of college students with trouble snoozing. Try these simple tips for a great night's sleep — without drugs.

- Make lavender essential oil part of your bedtime routine, perhaps in your bath or sprinkled on your pillowcase.

- Limit daytime naps to 20 or 30 minutes.

- Steer clear of food and drinks, like coffee, that could keep you up at night.

- Stick to a regular bedtime routine.

- Keep your bedroom cool — between 60 and 67 degrees.

- Power down electronics with bright screens.

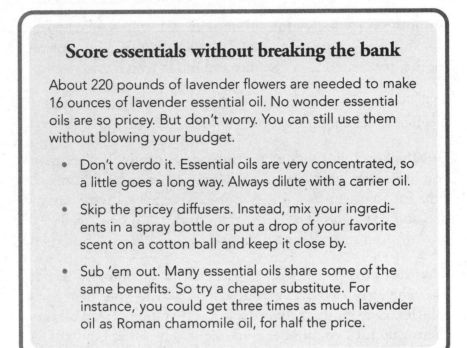

Score essentials without breaking the bank

About 220 pounds of lavender flowers are needed to make 16 ounces of lavender essential oil. No wonder essential oils are so pricey. But don't worry. You can still use them without blowing your budget.

- Don't overdo it. Essential oils are very concentrated, so a little goes a long way. Always dilute with a carrier oil.

- Skip the pricey diffusers. Instead, mix your ingredients in a spray bottle or put a drop of your favorite scent on a cotton ball and keep it close by.

- Sub 'em out. Many essential oils share some of the same benefits. So try a cheaper substitute. For instance, you could get three times as much lavender oil as Roman chamomile oil, for half the price.

3 ways essential oils bring out your natural beauty

Who IS that in the mirror? And where did those wrinkles come from? If you've recently been surprised by some sneaky signs of aging, you've come to the right place. Essential oils pack everything you need to rejuvenate your body from head to toe.

Save face with regenerating oils. Usually you're fine with being called mature. But when it comes to your skin, mature is the last word you want to hear. Add these essential oils to your anti-aging arsenal to make wrinkles a thing of the past — frankincense, sweet fennel, and clary sage.

When applying any essential oil to your skin, remember to use a carrier oil. Jojoba oil does wonders because it's similar to sebum, a natural oil produced by your pores. Your skin soaks it up, softening lines and chasing away wrinkles.

Smooth on remedies for softer skin. Ashy elbows, itchy legs, cracking feet — dry skin can hit you at any time. To soften and soothe, try chamomile, jasmine, and sandalwood.

Make your own moisturizer by adding any of these to carrier oils like sweet almond, avocado, or coconut oil.

Get thicker, fuller hair with drug-free therapy. If it seems you have more hair in your comb than on your head, it may be time for an essential oil intervention. Rosemary, thyme, lavender, and cedarwood encourage scalp health and boost hair growth. And researchers have a study to back it up.

They recruited people with alopecia areata, an autoimmune disease where your body's immune system attacks your hair follicles. One group massaged jojoba oil and grapeseed oil into their scalp for two minutes every night. The other group did the same, except their mixture also contained essential oils. After seven months, three times as many people treated with this aromatic mixture reported positive results compared to those in the group that used no essential oils.

Want to give it a go? Try this recipe.

Essential oils:

- 3 drops lavender oil
- 3 drops rosemary oil
- 2 drops cedarwood oil
- 2 drops thyme oil

Carrier oils:

- 1 teaspoon jojoba oil
- 4 teaspoons grapeseed oil

Fermented foods

Gut check: fight tummy troubles with fermented fare

While fermentation may seem new and trendy, it's actually been around for thousands of years. Take fruit, vegetables, grains, meat, or even milk, throw in some bacteria or yeast, allow it to sit long enough to undergo a chemical change, and, voilà, you end up with something different in flavor and texture. A food that is naturally preserved to last longer than it would otherwise. A food that is often healthier because it contains new compounds or because its nutrients are more available.

In some cases, fermentation was discovered by accident. Here are some early examples.

- Herdsmen in ancient Asia stored the milk from their animals in containers without refrigeration. Eventually, the natural enzymes in the milk curdled it, breaking it down chemically, turning it thick and sour. This process also produced lactic acid, which acts as a preservative, helping the fermented milk stay fresh longer. The result — yogurt.

- In hot, sunny climates, people used to dry meat to make it store better. But in areas like northern Europe, they needed a different method. So they turned to curing. By salting, spicing, and smoking ground meat, they were able to keep sausages at room temperature for up to 40 days after cutting. The beneficial organisms introduced during this process prevent the destructive or toxic ones from growing, so the meat doesn't spoil.

- The word sauerkraut is German, meaning "sour cabbage." But the food probably originated in China over 2,000 years ago when laborers ate fermented shredded cabbage as they built the Great Wall. Immerse vegetables like cucumbers, beets, cauliflower, radishes, onions, peppers, or cabbage in salt or vinegar, and lactic microbial organisms develop. These turn the food's natural sugars into lactic acid. Now the harmful bacteria that cause spoilage can't multiply.

> Unlike healthy fermented fare, highly salted foods are some of the most dangerous for your bowel, because they are associated with a greater risk of stomach cancer. Don't overindulge in pickled items for this reason. One exception — miso soup. The soy in it seems to cancel out the harmful effects of its salt.

Fermented and fabulous. Curdling milk, curing meats, and pickling vegetables are all types of fermentation. And a surprise bonus — if the foods are not cooked or exposed to high heat, they still contain live, friendly bacteria, called probiotics, that deliver amazing health benefits.

The International Scientific Association for Probiotics and Prebiotics (ISAPP) says fermented foods are valuable because they:

- are a source of live, active microbes.

- improve taste and texture, and make foods easier to digest.

- increase concentrations of vitamins and other beneficial compounds in foods.

- remove or reduce toxins in raw foods.

- increase food safety and shelf life.

Shop like a pro for probiotics. Some fermented foods are further processed, perhaps by pasteurization, baking, canning, or filtering. This kills the active microbes. That's why many popular fermented foods lack probiotics.

So that jar of pickles on the supermarket shelf is without good gut bugs, because it's been pasteurized. But the jar in the refrigerated aisle may be just what you're looking for. Keep an eye out for these labels — raw, unpasteurized, or live active cultures — if you want a product with probiotics.

Fermented foods with living cultures	Fermented foods without living cultures
fresh kimchi	chocolate
fresh sauerkraut	most beer
fresh sour pickles	most soy sauce
kefir	most wine
miso	sourdough bread
some cheeses	tempeh
traditional salami	
water- or brine-cured olives	
yogurt	

Gut bugs take the bite out of belly maladies. As you eat fermented fare with active probiotics, something incredible happens. Your GI tract fills up with millions of microbes that maintain your gut's health and harmony. That's not all. Studies show these amazing gut bugs prevent or help heal the following:

- irritable bowel syndrome (IBS)
- ulcerative colitis
- colon cancer
- diarrhea
- lactose intolerance
- stomach ulcers

How bacteria put up their dukes. That's quite a list, isn't it? What's even more remarkable is how battle-ready strains of bacteria like *Lactobacillus* and *Bifidobacteria* — the very probiotics in many fermented foods — fight for your health. Probiotics:

- lower the pH in your intestines, creating an environment toxic to harmful bugs.

- boost substances called mucins that protect you from bad bacteria.

- stimulate and strengthen your immune system.

- block bad bugs from getting out of your intestines and into your bloodstream, which lowers your risk of infections and food allergies.

Special K KO's 3 deadly diseases

Browse the vitamin aisle and you'll find something for anything that ails you. One nutrient clobbers colds while another makes your skin look younger. But what if you could find a vitamin that tackles heart disease, osteoporosis, and cancer? Reach for vitamin K — the one vitamin that can help prevent them all.

While it's not risen to celebrity status, like C or D, vitamin K is as essential as cool water on a hot summer day. Scrape a knee, for instance, and K comes to the rescue. This trusty nutrient helps your blood clot at the site so you won't bleed to death.

Vitamin K breaks down into two main forms:

- K1 or phylloquinone is found in green veggies like kale and broccoli, and in certain plant oils, like canola and soybean.

- K2 or menaquinone is produced by bacteria in your digestive system. But you can also find it in certain fermented foods like cheese, butter, cottage cheese, and a fermented soybean dish called natto. With a mild, earthy flavor, natto is actually the richest food source of K2. However, the slimy texture makes it an acquired taste. Tame it by serving over rice in true Japanese fashion.

Your body needs both K1 and K2, but if you're worried about the following age-related diseases, make K2 your go-to. It tackles the most jobs in your body and is without question the more powerful antioxidant.

> Store fermented foods at 115 degrees or cooler. High heat zaps all those wonderful gut bugs. Cold temps, and even freezing, does not.

Heart disease. The famous Rotterdam study followed close to 5,000 healthy men and women for up to 10 years, and showed those getting the most K2 had a 41 percent lower risk of heart disease. K2 works by keeping your blood vessels flexible and blocking the buildup of dangerous calcium deposits.

Osteoporosis. K2 lowers your chances of suffering hip, spine, and all other fractures by strengthening your bones. In fact, some doctors already prescribe a daily dose of 45 milligrams (mg) of K2 to treat osteoporosis.

Cancer. Two clinical trials found 45 mg of K2 a day blocked the growth of liver cancer in people with existing liver damage. And it put the brakes on liver cancer coming back. Scientists believe K2 works by activating proteins that stop cancer cells from growing.

Surprising cause of allergy symptoms

Watch out. Fermented foods are chock-full of a substance called histamine. And if you're an allergy sufferer, you're well aware of the havoc histamines wreak in your body — itchy eyes, a runny nose, hives, congestion, headaches, and a slew of other uncomfortable symptoms.

What's more, mold and yeast are part of the fermentation process. They can also trigger allergy-like symptoms.

If you react after eating fermented foods, don't think this means you're allergic to them. It means you have a food "intolerance." The symptoms are similar, but it doesn't involve your immune system.

What's good for the gut is good for the gray matter

What you eat can keep you sharp and stress-free. Researchers have been studying the connection between your belly and your brain, and they've come to a delicious conclusion. Fermented foods benefit both.

Eat to keep your memories from fading. Think better and remember more with these two tasty ways to protect your brain.

- Vinegar is not only a fermented food, itself, but is also used to ferment other foods, thanks to its heaping helping of acetic acid bacteria (AAB). And it is AAB that triggers your body to produce special building blocks for brain tissue called sphingolipids. These are essential for specialized nerve cells to function properly. Without the right balance of sphingolipids, your risk of conditions like Alzheimer's disease (AD) increases.

- Cheese, like camembert, is fermented with the bacteria *Penicillium candidum*, and produces an organic compound called oleamide. This blocks brain inflammation and reduces the buildup of amyloid plaques, a telltale sign of AD. Scientists say camembert alone won't prevent dementia, but eating it as part of a well-balanced meal plan, like the Mediterranean diet, could help.

Probiotics help you chill out. Social anxiety. It's a stuffy term for the third largest mental health problem in the world today. You suffer from it if you dread interacting with people, often feel insecure or embarrassed around others, and generally believe you are always being watched and judged.

So how could fermented foods possibly help this emotional roller coaster? "It is likely that the probiotics in fermented foods are favorably changing the environment in the gut," says psychology professor Matthew Hilimire, "and changes in the gut in turn influence social anxiety."

Probiotics reduce activity in brain areas involved in reacting to negative social situations and may regulate a natural substance called gamma-aminobutyric acid (GABA). Much like anti-anxiety pills, GABA helps to control fear and anxiety when neurons become overexcited. In other words, it calms the jitters.

People who ate more fermented foods — like yogurt, kefir, miso soup, sauerkraut, pickles, tempeh, and kimchi — felt less stressed in social situations like speaking in public or meeting strangers, found an American research team. Those prone to feeling higher levels of fear and worry benefitted the most.

Fish oil

Heart problems? Fish oil to the rescue

A pill that can help you recover from heart attack and stroke sounds too amazing to be true. After all, many so-called miracle cures turn out to be completely bogus.

But this isn't snake oil — it's fish oil. Two supplements a day will give you the same omega-3 fatty acids as two servings of fish a week. That could help you ward off heart problems — and depression, diabetes, and cancer, to boot. If you think these claims sound a bit fishy, don't worry — evidence shows these nutrient-packed pills actually work.

Omega-3 fatty acids can heal your heart. Everybody has their go-to cure for a broken heart — some people listen to country music, and others dig into a big tub of ice cream. But if your heart literally needs a tune-up, grab a bottle of fish oil.

In a new study, researchers in Boston discovered high-dose fish oil supplements will actually help your heart heal itself after a heart attack. Over the course of six months, subjects who took omega-3 supplements had less scarring and thickening in their hearts than those who didn't take omega-3. Even better, their hearts pumped blood more efficiently.

Participants in the study took 4 grams of prescription fish oil every day. But over-the-counter supplements are not as regulated, so don't take high doses without talking to your doctor.

Kick-start your stroke recovery with fish oil. In the past, experts thought fish oil supplements could help lower your chances of stroke. But now experts aren't so sure. In fact, new studies show that supplements might not affect your risk of stroke at all.

But that doesn't mean you should throw in the towel on fish oil just yet. High doses of fish oil may be just what your body needs after suffering from one of these dreaded attacks.

> Fish oil supplements are not for everyone. When taken with blood thinners or high blood pressure medicines, they may increase the effects of the medication. That could result in dangerous, even fatal, side effects. Talk to your doctor before taking this supplement.

A new animal study discovered that omega-3 fatty acids can start repairing damaged brain cells after a stroke. Experts think this could help stroke sufferers improve their motor function and avoid long-term brain damage.

Results look promising, but it still needs to be tested on people. Stay tuned.

Turn to DHA to keep cancer at bay

You may think omega-3 fatty acids are all the same, but that's not the case. Omega-3 breaks down into two major categories.

- Short chain acids, like alpha-linolenic acid (ALA), come from plants and nuts.

- Long chain acids, like eicosapentaenoic acid (EPA) and docosahexaenoic acid (DHA), are found in fatty fish and some algaes.

Each has a different number of carbon atoms, not to mention different, tongue-twisting names! Their small distinctions may not seem important, but they are when it comes to fighting disease. For example, scientists have discovered that one particular fatty acid — DHA — may be the key to warding off cancer.

A group of Italian researchers recently found that DHA targets and attacks multiple myeloma cells, causing them to die. Other studies have found that DHA can stop colon tumors from forming. It works by blocking the growth of cancer cells and triggering their death.

Cancer research on fatty acids is still in its early stages. But if you want to give yourself a leg up, focus on eating more foods with omega-3. Salmon is your best option for DHA. A 3-ounce serving has more than 1,000 milligrams of DHA — up to 15 times more than other seafood.

> The fatty acids in fish oil may fight cancer but, unfortunately, they attack cancer fighters, too. Recent studies discovered that a specific fatty acid in fish oil lowers the effectiveness of chemotherapy. So it's best to avoid using fish oil or eating fatty fish during treatment.

If you prefer, you can take a DHA supplement or fish oil with both DHA and EPA. Experts say it's safe to get up to 4 grams of fish oil daily. But if you're considering taking a supplement, talk to your doctor first.

Scale up your protection to take on diabetes

Fighting diabetes requires all-out effort. This disease affects some 30 million Americans, with more than a million new cases diagnosed every year. So if you want to come out on top, you'll need all the protection you can get. Fish oil is one power-ful, natural armor you should consider adding to your arsenal.

Omega-3 fatty acids keep insulin in check. Keeping your blood sugar balanced will help you get a leg up on diabetes. And experts think fish oil may be a key to doing just that.

In a study published in *The Journal of Clinical Endocrinology and Metabolism*, researchers reviewed clinical trials that focused on omega-3 fatty acids and their effect on a protein hormone called adiponectin. This naturally occurring hormone has pow-erful anti-inflammatory properties and can improve your body's sensitivity to insulin. That helps keep your blood sugar stable.

The researchers discovered that omega-3 fatty acids help fight diabetes by increasing your body's production of adiponectin. Previous studies have shown that the more adiponectin in your bloodstream, the lower your risk of type 2 diabetes.

Soothe your nerves and save your sight with this fishy delight. It's never too late to start enjoying the benefits of fish oil. Even if you already suffer from diabetes, the powerful nutri-ents can help you dodge dangerous complications.

- Diabetic neuropathy. High blood sugar can cause tingling, numbness, and if left untreated, permanent nerve damage. In a new animal study, researchers from the University of Iowa found the omega-3 fatty acids in fish oil can help pre-vent this damage. And a compound in fish oil called resolvin actually stimulates the regrowth of damaged nerves.

"Even though a lot more work needs to be done, including clinical trials with human subjects, our animal studies sug-gest that fish oil can reverse some of the harmful effects of diabetes on the nerves," says lead researcher Mark Yorek.

- Diabetic retinopathy. Getting at least 500 milligrams of omega-3 every day can protect your eyes from this sight-threatening condition, studies show. You'll get more than enough simply by eating 3 ounces of salmon twice a week. High blood sugar can cause tiny blood vessels in your eyes to swell and leak, eventually leading to vision loss and even permanent blindness. But experts think the powerful anti-inflammatory effects of fish oil can help protect your blood vessels and lower your risk of vision loss.

Reel in the facts — which supplement is right for you?

Fish oil pills are loaded with docosahexaenoic acid (DHA) and eicosapentaenoic acid (EPA), but they aren't the only options on the market.

- Krill oil supplements are a great way to amp up your EPA intake. They are made from tiny crustaceans rather than fatty fish, and are often higher in EPA.

- Omega-3 fatty acids from algae are a great vegetarian option, but they often offer only DHA. You may have to get EPA from another source. Fortunately, your body can turn alpha-linolenic acid (ALA) from plant foods, like walnuts and flaxseed, into EPA.

A promising way to lift the veil of depression

Getting over depression is not like fighting the flu. Your body may not get better on its own. Clinical depression is a disease but not one caused by bacteria or viruses. Instead, it's caused by an imbalance of chemicals in your brain.

To fight off major depression, doctors often prescribe antidepressants to get your brain back on track. But sometimes it's not enough. People can take several courses of antidepressants and still not feel better.

That's where fish oil comes in. A recent review of 13 studies revealed that omega-3 supplements actually boost the effectiveness of prescription antidepressants. Researchers think it's the eicosapentaenoic acid (EPA) in fish oil that's responsible for the mood-boosting effects. They aren't quite sure why but think it may have something to do with EPA's ability to fight inflammation.

Studies have shown you can take up to 1,000 milligrams of EPA a day. If you can't find it as a single supplement, simply take a regular fish oil supplement that contains EPA. Scientists thought the docosahexaenoic acid (DHA) in fish oil might counteract the protective effects of EPA, but tests showed that wasn't the case.

Taking these supplements along with antidepressants isn't known to cause any major side effects, but you should still talk to your doctor before trying fish oil.

Flaxseed

Tiny seeds pose a triple threat to your biggest health woes

King Charlemagne was so taken with flaxseed, he passed laws requiring his subjects to eat it. While the health claims may have been hard to swallow in the eighth century, today scientists agree flaxseed helps protect against three of your biggest health concerns — weight gain, rising blood sugar levels, and heart disease. This superfood does it all.

Pack on the flax, not the pounds. Watching the scale go up year after year can get you down. But flaxseed has a secret weapon — lignans. These plant estrogens mimic hormones that help regulate body weight.

The magic starts in your gut where bacteria convert plant lignans into compounds your body can use to control the formation of fat tissue. Researchers recently discovered women who ate more foods containing lignans weighed less and had less belly fat, compared to women eating fewer lignan-rich foods. In fact, they gained about half a pound less each year.

And it doesn't stop there. When your digestive system breaks down the fiber in flax, your body produces hormones that make you feel fuller and more satisfied. The upshot — you eat less and like your scale more.

Fill up with fiber to balance blood sugar. You may associate the phrase "sugar rush" with your 10th birthday party, but if your blood sugar levels are constantly too high, you may be putting future birthdays in jeopardy. Flaxseed again delivers the gift of fiber, which balances your blood sugar.

Fiber is a particularly underappreciated part of the American diet. In fact, most people only get about half of the recommended amount. Which is a shame because soluble fiber helps slow digestion, lowering the amount of sugar that makes it to your bloodstream.

To see if flax would hit the mark, people with pre-diabetes added about two tablespoons of ground flaxseed to their daily diets. That's about 4 grams of extra fiber a day. After three months, flax significantly improved how their bodies responded to insulin.

Flax: the eggless baking fix

Whether you're dealing with egg allergies, trying to stick to a vegan diet, or looking for ways to bump up your daily flax intake, keep this neat trick up your sleeve, and you'll be the best baker in the kitchen.

For every egg in your recipe, substitute a mixture of 1 tablespoon ground flaxseed and 3 tablespoons water. Let the combo sit for about 10 minutes to thicken. You're on your way to baking delicious egg-free cookies, waffles, muffins, and more.

Set your heart on healing with ALA. Alpha-linolenic acid (ALA) is a kind of omega-3 fatty acid found in plants like flaxseed. It's famous for lowering inflammation, LDL cholesterol, and other heart disease risk factors, like high blood pressure. Want proof?

People in one study ate foods like muffins and bagels every day containing about four tablespoons of ground flaxseed. After six months, their systolic blood pressure dropped 10 points, which could cut stroke risk by 36 percent and risk of heart attacks by 27 percent.

Latest on lignans — beat breast cancer from your pantry

No way itty-bitty brown seeds can hold a candle to cutting-edge breast cancer preventive strategies, right? Maybe — if those seeds are packed with lifesaving lignans, a type of plant nutrient similar to the hormone estrogen.

To understand why, you need to look at your body through a microscope.

Each cell in your body has a nucleus that acts as a control center and includes instructions for the cell. When cells get worn out or damaged, they copy these instructions to new cells that take their place.

Unfortunately, cells sometimes misread these instructions. They go places they aren't supposed to. They ignore emergency protocol and don't die when they're damaged. They can also divide and create more abnormal cells. This is called cancer. Estrogen often plays a role in breast cancer because it can attach to estrogen receptors in breast cells and encourage them to grow — even the cancerous ones.

Enter lignans. With a chemical structure similar to your own estrogen, they compete for space on cells. But they don't send the same message as estrogen. This may be one of the ways they discourage the spread of cancer, say scientists who have the studies to back it up.

- Young women who were already at high risk for breast cancer took lignan supplements for a year. The verdict — Ki-67, a substance associated with cancer growth, went down in 80 percent of the women. That means fewer precancerous changes. Experts say you may get similar benefits with a daily teaspoon of ground flaxseed.

- In another study, breast cancer patients ate a muffin containing about four tablespoons of ground flaxseed each day. In five weeks, flax helped slow cell growth and remove unhealthy cells. It even changed the characteristics of the cancer cells to a less aggressive form.

This super seed has lignan levels up to 800 times higher than many other plant foods. That makes flaxseed a natural, side effect-free way to lower your risk of breast cancer.

Oil up with flax for relief in the palm of your hand

If you have numb, tingling palms or wrist pain, listen up. In a stroke of genius, scientists decided to test flaxseed oil on the symptoms of carpal tunnel syndrome. And guess what? It worked.

This condition is no stranger to many who labor all day on a computer or assembly line, or suffer from arthritis, diabetes, or several other conditions. They all cause pressure on your median nerve. This bundle of sensory fibers runs from your forearm to your hand, through a narrow opening in your wrist, called the carpal tunnel. When the carpal tunnel narrows, your median nerve is squeezed, and you feel it in your fingers, palm, wrist, and arm.

People with carpal tunnel syndrome rubbed 5 drops of flaxseed oil on their problem wrist two times a day and wore a wrist splint at night. Within a month, symptoms improved by 30 percent. Imagine being able to cook, sew, or garden again without wrist discomfort or weakness.

Then researchers out of Iran compared just flaxseed oil gel to wrist splints. And surprise, the flax was more effective. Some scientists chalk it up to nutrients like alpha-linolenic acid (ALA). These omega-3s help block inflammation and relieve pain.

If you want to give it a go, talk to your doctor to see what flaxseed product may be right for you.

Season cast iron to perfection with secret flax fix

A hard, slick surface and a dark sheen is the mark of cast iron perfection. But if your traditional seasoning methods aren't getting you there, try this flaxseed oil trick that's been praised by cookware designers and professional test kitchens.

- Warm your pan in a 200-degree oven for about 15 minutes to open up the pores of the iron.

- Carefully remove the pan, pour in a dab of organic, 100-percent flaxseed oil, and rub it into every inch of the surface. Use paper or cotton towels to wipe off any excess oil, so the pan looks dry.

- Turn the pan upside down in the oven, and set the temperature to 500 degrees, or as hot as it goes.

- Once your oven reaches this temp, heat your pan for one hour. Then turn off the oven, and let the pan cool for two hours.

- Take the pan out, and repeat the oiling, heating, and cooling process five more times.

Gelatin

Gelatin gets your joints jumping

Strawberry, raspberry, or cherry. With a dollop of whipped topping. Do you remember trying to guess the flavor of that jiggly red dessert when you were a kid? Well, this is not exactly your grandmother's jello. But Granny might have had a little more spring in her step — and less creak in her knees — if she'd just added some gelatin to her daily diet. Not the sugary red stuff, though. The plain, unsweetened kind is best for your joints. Gelatin for joints? You bet.

Go crazy for collagen. To understand gelatin, you have to first understand collagen. It's the protein found in many animals, including humans. In fact, collagen makes up almost a third of the protein in your body. Its job is to strengthen connective tissues, like cartilage, ligaments, and tendons.

Centuries ago, people boiled animal skins, bones, and hooves to produce a jelly-like substance. What they were really doing was releasing the collagen. You've probably experienced this yourself. Simmer meat bones for soup, chill it, and you'll end up with a congealed broth. And that's essentially how commercial gelatin is prepared today, from cow bones and hides, pork skins and bones, chicken bones, and — for some kosher products — fish skins.

The end result, basically cooked collagen, is odorless, tasteless, and colorless. After processing, it's used by food manufacturers as a binder and a thickening agent in lots of products, from bouillon to yogurt, marshmallows to canned ham. And, oh yes, in jiggly desserts.

A dynamic duo for your joints. With age, your body produces less collagen. Those achy knees? Right. Less collagen means less cartilage and stiffer joints. But, with a little help from vitamin C, the collagen in gelatin may boost your body's natural collagen enough to make you more flexible.

A new study, published in the *American Journal of Clinical Nutrition*, explained how volunteers drank up to three teaspoons of a gelatin supplement with added vitamin C. After an hour, they performed six minutes of high-impact exercise — jumping rope — to rev up the collagen-building compounds in their joints. They did this three times a day for three days.

> The gelatin that eases your achy knees could soothe painful joints for your dog or cat. First, check with your vet to see how much gelatin you should add to your pet's meal. Then make sure you buy a plain, unsweetened brand that's free from artificial colors or flavors. Additives like those could do more harm than good.

Then researchers tested their blood for amino acids associated with building collagen. They found these important markers had doubled.

Bottom line? There's evidence a gelatin and vitamin C combo boosts your body's production of collagen, which can mean healthier ligaments and bones, less pain and stiffness in joints, and better mobility for arthritis sufferers.

Kitchen notes:
there's always room for gelatin

Powdered, unflavored gelatin has no sugar or other additives. Which means you can use it in sweet or savory dishes. Here are two great ideas to get you started.

- Turn thin store-bought stock into rich, silky pan sauce or gravy with better flavor and texture. Simply sprinkle 1 1/2 teaspoons of gelatin onto 1 cup of stock and set it aside for a few minutes. Once the powder is absorbed, stir the stock into your pan and heat as usual.

- Concoct your own gelatin-vitamin C powerhouse with a refreshing fruit salad. Prepare unflavored gelatin as instructed using water or fruit juice. Include a little lemon and sugar to taste. Allow to thicken slightly in the fridge. Stir in fresh strawberries.

Your 'key' to better bones

A 12-month study at Florida State University tested the effectiveness of a calcium-collagen chelate — pronounced "key-late" — in women with low bone density. This condition, called osteopenia, can lead to fragile bones and an increased risk for fracture.

Half the women in the study took 5 grams of a compound containing calcium and collagen bound together. The supplement also included vitamin D. The remaining women took the same amount of calcium and vitamin D only.

The calcium-collagen chelate set lost a little over 1 percent in bone density during the year, while the other group lost almost 4 percent.

Collagen 2 ways: clearing up the confusion

To get raw collagen, you'd have to sit around gnawing on bones or, in a slightly more civilized fashion, drink bone broth. The latter has its own set of health issues, including the risk of lead contamination. Thank goodness you have other ways to add collagen to your diet — gelatin and collagen hydrolysate, also called hydrolyzed collagen.

Both contain the same amino acids and both come in powdered form or as capsules. Collagen hydrolysate, however, is more processed than gelatin, with its proteins broken down into tinier bits. While the main difference between the two is how quickly they are absorbed in your body, they also vary in other ways, including how you can use them in your kitchen.

Gelatin	Collagen hydrolysate
May cause digestive problems in some people	Processed into smaller proteins, so more easily absorbed
Only dissolves in hot water	Dissolves in both hot and cold water
Causes liquids to gel	Does not gel
Used to thicken soups or sauces	Great added to smoothies
Supplements may be unsafe in high doses	Talk to your doctor before using protein powders for weight loss

Face up to wrinkles with collagen

"With mirth and laughter let old wrinkles come," penned William Shakespeare in *The Merchant of Venice.* But once those wrinkles start coming, it's hard to slow them down. You might need a little collagen in your corner.

Face facts. Collagen forms a network of cells in the middle layer of your skin where new cells can grow. And it helps replace and restore dead skin cells while it keeps your skin strong and smooth. But your body's collagen production starts declining pretty fast beginning in your 20s — around 1 percent a year. It continues to nosedive in your 40s and 50s, followed by a 30-percent plummet in the first few years after menopause. Add that to all those summers spent in the sun, and it's no wonder those crow's feet are marching across your face.

Can collagen plump you up? Collagen molecules are too big to pass through the skin's surface, so creams may not be your best option. Some experts think a better way to get your collagen is to just take a drink. Of hydrolyzed collagen, that is. Also called collagen peptide, it has been processed so that the molecules are smaller and more easily absorbed by your system.

In a German study of over 100 women ages 45 to 65, participants took either a placebo or a mixture containing bioactive collagen peptide (BCP) every day for eight weeks. The women who drank the BCP noticed fewer wrinkles around their eyes. And the improvements in their skin's moisture and elasticity lasted for four weeks after they stopped taking the supplement.

Are you ready to go head-to-head with those smile lines? Products like these are trendy — and can be expensive. While current research seems to support drinkable collagen, for the argument to be truly convincing, more and better clinical trials need to be done.

Ginger

This common spice leads the crackdown on cholesterol

You wouldn't dream of pouring mud into your car's oil tank. The thick sludge would clog every hose and pipe in the engine. And you'd have to take one expensive trip to the mechanic. So why would you let cholesterol do the same thing to you? When you pump your body full of fatty foods, you're gumming up your veins and arteries. And if you're not careful, this can lead to hardened blood vessels, blood clots, strokes, and heart attacks.

Perhaps you already stick to a healthy diet, but remember, even a Ferrari needs a tune-up every now and then. Ginger could be the key to keeping your pipes clean. This spice works hard to stop cholesterol from slowing you down.

Saudi Arabian researchers recently pitted ginger's powers against a placebo pill. After only 45 days, people who took ginger had much lower LDL cholesterol than those who didn't.

Experts believe certain compounds in ginger keep you from absorbing too much cholesterol and fat from the foods you eat.

People in this study took 3 grams of powdered ginger a day. If you want to try this at home, that works out to be about 1 1/2 teaspoons. While ginger is considered safe, taking this much might cause an upset stomach or heartburn.

Lowering your cholesterol isn't the only thing ginger is good for. Read on to learn how it can wake up your immune system and work as a natural anti-inflammatory.

Doubling down with ginger spells danger

Ginger is a great way to strike back against high cholesterol and protect your heart, but it doesn't always mix well with prescription drugs. If you're taking a blood-thinning medication like warfarin (Coumadin), ginger could have dangerous side effects.

This spicy spice also works to slow down blood clotting — just like prescription drugs. While this helps you avoid heart attacks and strokes, you can have too much of a good thing. Adding supplements or large amounts of ginger to your diet could cause excessive bruising or bleeding.

Soothe inflammation to crush a triple threat

Cancer, arthritis, and allergies might sound like a strange trio, but something surprising ties these chronic conditions together — inflammation.

Normally, your body uses inflammation to keep germs, pollutants, and other irritants in check. However, sometimes signals get crossed. When that happens, inflammation can trigger everything from colon cancer to hay fever. If you want to get ahead of these conditions, look for a little help from one of nature's best inflammation fighters — ginger.

This spicy treat curbs your risk of cancer. Greasy, fried foods might be your guilty pleasure, but they put you at risk of colon cancer. Items fried in polyunsaturated oils, like corn, safflower, and soybean, cause your body to create compounds called eicosanoids.

In small amounts, eicosanoids are actually healthy. But if you go overboard, they trigger inflammation which can lead to cancer.

A study published in *Cancer Prevention Research* revealed ginger has the power to rein in this process by keeping your body from turning fatty acids into eicosanoids.

People in this study took a ginger extract, equal to a whopping 20 grams of raw ginger, every day for 28 days. That's a lot — almost 3 1/2 tablespoons. Talk to your doctor before taking this amount of ginger, since it can cause heartburn or upset stomach in some people.

Put knee pain in the past with a natural anti-inflammatory. Aching joints make everyday tasks seem impossible. But adding a dash of ginger to your homemade smoothies will have you back in action in no time. Studies show ginger is a safe and effective way to thwart painful inflammation caused by knee arthritis.

Experts recommend adding just a half-teaspoon of powdered ginger to your daily diet. Get creative and throw a bit of ginger into your next curry or stir-fry for an extra kick.

Breathe easy — compounds in ginger fight back against allergies. Your immune system works hard to protect your body from dangerous germs, but sometimes it goes a little too far. It starts to think things like dust, fur, or pollen are deadly diseases, and triggers inflammation as a way to deal with them. According to animal studies, ginger blocks the messengers your body uses to trigger allergy symptoms.

This hasn't been tested on humans yet, so there's no recommended dose. But keep an eye out for more information.

Ditch the spice rack — your ginger belongs in the freezer

How often do you buy fresh ginger only to throw it away a few weeks later because it's wrinkled and dried out? A jar of the powdered stuff may be convenient, but has fewer active compounds than fresh. The answer is to stick that knobby root in the freezer. Here are the benefits:

- Frozen, it will last for at least six months. If you simply store it in the fridge, it will stay good for only about a month.

- It will be a breeze to grate. Room temperature or even chilled ginger leaves stubborn strings and pulp behind. But frozen ginger washes off your grater without a fuss.

And if the ginger in your freezer turns blue or gray, don't worry. Cold environments cause the natural plant chemicals in ginger, called anthocyanins, to turn blue. It might look moldy, but it's safe to eat.

2 ways to heat up your weight loss

A spice that burns calories? Not so crazy. Especially when there's science to back it up. Here are two ways a dash of ginger could melt away the pounds.

- Light a fire under your metabolism. According to a recent study published in the *European Journal of Nutrition*, ginger helps your body burn calories faster and more efficiently. Half the women in this study took 2 grams of ginger powder — about one heaping teaspoon — every day for three months. After 12 weeks, those in the ginger group had a significantly lower body mass index (BMI) than when they started, compared to those who took a placebo. Your BMI, remember, is a ratio of your weight to your height, and is considered a good gauge of body fat.

- Don't fret the fat. Pizza and burgers are hard to resist, but these fatty foods always leave you feeling guilty. Fortunately, ginger might help ease your mind after the occasional indulgence. According to an animal study, this spice helps block your gut from absorbing too much fat from the food you eat.

All-natural miracle fix for your migraine

Shimmering lights flood your vision. Everything seems a little too loud and a little too bright. If you suffer from migraines, you know exactly what's coming. You could turn to drugs to keep the headaches at bay, but most put you at risk of vertigo, dizziness, and even heart attacks. Great news — there's a safer, cheaper cure hidden in your pantry.

The next time you feel a migraine coming on, reach for some ginger. According to a recent study, one-eighth teaspoon of powdered ginger can treat the crippling pain as well as leading drugs.

Ginger works by fighting off natural hormones called prostaglandins which trigger painful inflammation in blood vessels during a migraine.

Here are some ideas that will have you turning to the spice rack instead of the medicine cabinet.

- Simmer a few peeled, thinly sliced pieces of fresh ginger in hot water. Let steep for 10 minutes, remove the ginger, and enjoy. For a strong, spicy tea, use more ginger, approximately 2 inches sliced, and simmer longer, for 20 minutes. Add honey or lime juice to taste.

- Juice or grate fresh ginger and add to sparkling mineral water or club soda. Pour over ice and — presto — genuine, homemade ginger ale.

- For a healthy kick, shake powdered ginger into your iced tea, lemonade, or even coffee.

Spice up your grocery shopping with fresh ginger

Need a fresh tomato or banana? That's a task every shopper can handle. But choosing fresh ginger is a bit more challenging. Follow these tips and you'll take home fresh, flavorful ginger every time.

- Trust your nose. Fresh ginger smells spicy and strong. If you can't smell it, don't buy it.

- Twist and snap. Ginger grows in large roots, but you don't have to buy the whole chunk. Most stores let you break off what you need. If it's fresh, it should snap easily.

- Stay smooth. Wrinkled, rough ginger is over the hill. Look for shiny, smooth-skinned pieces instead.

Grapefruit

This fruit is ripe with heart-healthy benefits

One bite of this tropical delight can inspire dreams of sun-kissed shores. Even grapefruit's botanical name — *Citrus paradisi* — conjures up images of swaying palm trees and gentle ocean breezes. But this tart and tasty fruit is no watered-down weakling. It's packed with a heart-healthy compound that fights high blood pressure and dangerously stiff arteries. *Citrus paradisi*, indeed.

You can blame the natural compound naringin, a type of flavanone, for grapefruit's bitter taste. But you also have to give it a tip of the cap for keeping your blood pressure in check and your blood vessels healthy.

Naringin opens up your blood flow. It works by increasing the amount of nitric oxide (NO) in your blood. And that's good because superstar NO, proclaimed "Molecule of the Year" in 1992, makes your blood vessels dilate, allowing blood to flow more freely and lowering blood pressure.

In studies of more than 200 people, researchers concluded grapefruit's naringin was responsible for a significant drop in systolic blood pressure. This top number in your reading indicates how hard blood pushes against your artery walls when your heart beats.

Then Israeli researchers had people with high blood pressure drink two cups of a juice with boosted levels of naringin every day for five weeks. They reported in the *American Journal of Hypertension* diastolic readings dropped more than eight points.

This bottom number represents how hard your blood pushes against artery walls while your heart is resting between beats.

Flexible blood vessels are heart healthy. Half of the women in one French study drank grapefruit juice. The other half were given a similar juice with no flavanones. After six months, they switched. So what did researchers learn? Grapefruit's flavanones caused the women's blood vessels to be more flexible. And when it comes to blood vessels, the more flexible they are, the better the blood flow to your heart.

Grapefruit's not for every body. If your doctor has diagnosed you with high blood pressure, grapefruit — or its juice — may not be right for you because it can alter the way your blood pressure medication works. Check with your pharmacist or doctor about possible side effects.

Grapefruit's potassium performs a delicate dance with sodium that keeps your fluid levels balanced. Take in too much sodium and you retain fluids, which ups your blood pressure. But potassium helps your kidneys get rid of extra fluid and sodium, dropping your blood pressure back to normal. A delicious cup of grapefruit sections with juice delivers 9 percent of your daily potassium requirement.

Grapefruit galore: celebrate this citrus 3 ways

They may look alike on the outside, but each variety brings its own special health benefits to your table.

- White varieties contain more naringin than either the red or pink varieties.

- Pink and red grapefruit contain loads of beta carotene and lycopene, two carotenoids with antioxidant properties. The darker the fruit, the greater the carotenoid content.

Salt unlocks grapefruit's sweet secrets

You've probably sweetened up that tart breakfast treat with a spoonful or two of sugar. But have you tried adding a little salt instead? The unlikely pairing of grapefruit and salt took Americans by storm in the 1940s when the country was gearing up for war, and sugar was in short supply. "Grapefruit tastes sweeter with salt!" proclaimed a 1946 Morton Salt ad. But how does that work? In the mid-1990s, researchers tested the way people taste salt, bitter, and sweet. They discovered salt's ions block grapefruit's bitter compounds, like naringin, allowing the sweet to shine through.

For certain medications, grapefruit is the forbidden fruit

When the Reverend Griffith Hughes saw his first grapefruit in the 1700s while traveling in Barbados, he named it "The Forbidden Fruit." A man ahead of his time. Because if you're taking certain medications, you should avoid grapefruit and its juice — just like Adam should have dodged that apple.

Don't risk serious complications with your heart drugs.
Some medicines prescribed for the treatment of high cholesterol and high blood pressure are broken down in your small intestine by the enzyme CYP3A4, which controls how much of the drug makes it into your bloodstream.

Grapefruit and its juice contain compounds called furanocoumarins — a great word for Scrabble tournaments, but one that spells trouble for your medications. These furanocoumarins can block CYP3A4 from doing its work, causing your body to absorb too much medicine, and putting you at risk for health complications. These can range from mild muscle or joint pain to kidney failure.

- Statins for high cholesterol. According to doctors affiliated with the renowned Cleveland Clinic medical center and Harvard Medical School, you need to be especially concerned about the interaction of grapefruit products with these three statins — lovastatin (Mevacor), atorvastatin (Lipitor), and simvastatin (Zocor).

- Calcium channel blockers for high blood pressure. These drugs work by relaxing the muscles in the walls of your arteries. Avoid grapefruit if you take felodipine (Plendil) or nifedipine (Procardia and Adalat).

Grapefruit puts a hold on antihistamines. Some over-the-counter antihistamines like fexofenadine (Allegra) and diphenhydramine (Benadryl) reach your body's cells through proteins called transporters. Grapefruit can hinder the transporters from doing their job, which decreases the amount of medicine absorbed by your body. This makes the medicine less effective and you don't get the symptom relief you need.

But help for grapefruit lovers may be just over the horizon. Scientists are busy developing hybrid grapefruits that will be free of those bothersome furanocoumarins. Until then, check with your pharmacist or doctor before adding this "forbidden fruit" to your diet.

Freshen your home with some real a-peel

Is your bathtub grubby? Refrigerator rank? Kitchen faucet filmy? Scrub away stains and clear the air with these fresh 'n fruity tips.

Shine that grimy tub. The citric acid in grapefruit combined with coarse salt's scouring power make this a dynamic cleaning duo. Just cut your grapefruit in half and sprinkle it liberally with salt. Wet your bathtub and pour a little extra salt on the bottom of the tub. About one-fourth cup of salt for the whole job should do the trick. When you're finished scrubbing, simply rinse away the leftovers. All that remains is a spotless tub and the sweet citrus scent you love.

Put the sparkle back in your kitchen. Rub salt on a grapefruit half, scrub away at your water-stained faucet, then rinse. The salt and citric acid will work their magic, leaving behind nothing but shine.

Works for your glassware and silverware, or other surfaces like metal, porcelain, and glass. Grapefruit doesn't kill germs, though, so don't use it instead of dishwashing detergent.

Deodorize your smelly fridge. The squeezed-out leftovers from your morning grapefruit are perfect for this job. Slice the peel into pieces, place in a small bowl, and sprinkle with several tablespoons of salt. Place the bowl in your refrigerator, and let your grapefruit go to work. The next time you open your fridge, you'll be greeted with a fresh, citrusy fragrance.

Research shocker: grapefruit doesn't make you slim

Dieters put grapefruit to the test — and the fruit flunked. More than 200 overweight people either had a grapefruit product three times a day for up to 12 weeks — half a fresh grapefruit, about a cup of juice, or a grapefruit supplement — or they were part of the control group and had no grapefruit products at all. The results? The people in the grapefruit group lost no more weight than the controls.

Guava

Tropical treat — guard against cataracts with vitamin C

"C" is for cataract — a clouding of your lens that makes you feel like you're peering at the world through a foggy window. Luckily, you have another "C" that can combat blurry vision — vitamin C. Guavas have about four times the amount of vitamin C that oranges have, making them a delicious way to protect your peepers.

Oh, be careful little eyes what you see. Environmental factors like ultraviolet light can put your orbs in the danger zone by causing free radicals to form. These unpaired electrons like to couple up, so they scavenge the body, seeking out other electrons. This process, called oxidative stress, can harm your lenses, causing blurred vision, difficulty seeing at night, and light sensitivity.

But your body is prepared. The fluid that bathes your lenses contains vitamin C. This ordinary vitamin acts as an antioxidant, which is like a police force that steps in to stop the free radical riot.

Can eating more vitamin C protect your eyes? Scientists had to see for themselves, so they recruited 1,000 pairs of female twins and found two eye-opening results.

- Women who ate more vitamin C-rich foods had a 19-percent lower risk of cataracts, compared to those with diets low in this vision-saver.

- A decade later, researchers followed up with more than 300 pairs of the twins. Those who ate the most C were 33 percent less likely to experience cataract growth.

Experts say you may shrink cataract risk by eating more than 200 milligrams (mg) of vitamin C daily. Good news — it only takes a little guava to keep your vision sharp. One cup of the fruit contains a whopping 377 mg of nature's all-natural cataract preventer.

Taste tipoff: use your senses to serve guava at its peak

"You don't have to go all the way to Central America to get this exotic fruit," says Kimberly Lewis, who first tried guava juice and marmalade in Mexico. "I recently came across a container of guavas at my local Walmart." But how do you tell if your fruit is ready to eat?

- Touch. It should feel slightly soft.

- Sniff. You will smell a strong, sweet, musky fragrance.

- Look. The skin comes in various colors and often turns yellow, white, pink or light green when the fruit is ready to eat.

Ripe guavas don't last long, so eat up. Snack on them plain or add to fruit salads and smoothies. You can eat the skin and seeds. But be warned, guavas can host a bunch of hard seeds — up to 500. That's why many people prefer to rinse and slice the fruit, then scoop out the seeds.

3 ways guava beats out your biggest health worries

Cancer, heart disease, and bone loss. Oh my. This triple threat is your worst nightmare. You could turn to pills to guard your body. But how about a natural solution? Guava offers three-way protection in the form of an antioxidant called lycopene.

Here's the lowdown. Lycopene is a red pigment found in tomatoes, watermelon, papaya, and grapefruit. But if you're looking for the raw food that tops the charts, look no further than the humble guava.

Curb three types of cancer with one fruit. Lycopene acts as an antioxidant, which means it fends off free radicals that damage the building blocks of your body. In the case of cancer, it fights off toxins that can cause cell and DNA damage.

- Breast cancer. Women at a higher risk for breast cancer ate foods containing 25 milligrams (mg) of lycopene — equal to about 3 cups of guava fruit — every day. After 10 weeks, they had increased blood levels of adiponectin, a protein linked to lower breast cancer risk.

- Prostate cancer. The latest below-the-belt research comes from the Universities of Bristol, Cambridge, and Oxford. They found an 18-percent lower risk of prostate cancer in men who ate more than 10 servings of lycopene-rich foods each week.

- Kidney cancer. Scientists looked at the diets of more than 96,000 postmenopausal women enrolled in the Women's Health Initiative. Over the course of almost 20 years, those who reported eating more foods high in lycopene had a 39-percent lower risk of kidney cancer, compared to those who ate less.

Protect your ticker by targeting its biggest foes. Lycopene also makes sure your heart doesn't miss a beat. The antioxidant fights free radical damage, soothes inflammation, and lowers cholesterol. In addition, a review of several studies, published in the journal *Nutrients*, revealed the amount of lycopene found in about 1 1/2 cups of guava was enough to help reduce blood pressure.

Other studies show eating more lycopene-rich foods lowers your risk for heart disease and stroke. Less stress on your heart leads to a healthier you.

> More heartwarming news from the health front — guava has an amazing substance that washes artery-clogging LDL cholesterol right out of your body. At the same time, it raises the amount of good HDL cholesterol. What is it? Fiber. A cup of this delicious fruit contains about 36 percent of the fiber you need each day.

A few cups a day can beat brittle bones. Free radicals weaken your skeleton by damaging cells responsible for building and breaking down bone. Lycopene puts the kibosh on all that.

For four months, folks at the University of Toronto evaluated postmenopausal women who ate at least 30 mg of lycopene every day — the amount found in about 3 1/2 cups of guava fruit. Scientists noted a drop in N-telopeptide, a marker of bone breakdown closely linked to osteoporosis.

Wrinkle wars — shut down skin damage with a humble vitamin

Photodamage. No, it's not when your favorite family portrait starts to curl from spending one too many summers in the attic.

It happens when free radicals damage your skin, changing the structure and aging your appearance. The biggest culprit is ultraviolet (UV) light.

Exposure to UV rays can create too many free radical molecules in your skin. These trigger the breakdown of skin compounds like elastin and collagen, the connective tissues that keep your skin supple and wrinkle-free. That's like removing your skin's defense against wrinkles.

Of course, sunblock is a no-brainer. But for added protection, try some guava, the fruit that contains a nutrient proven to protect against aging skin — vitamin C.

Smooth sun-kissed skin with this antioxidant. Make no mistake, free radical damage isn't just going on behind the scenes. You and your mirror can often spot the side effects — roughness and discoloration.

Experts say vitamin C plays a big role in the skin renewal process. That's because it acts as an antioxidant to slash sun-related DNA and cell damage. Even when you give your skin a break from the sun, this powerful vitamin is still hard at work.

Cue collagen to fight fine lines. In addition to its antioxidant abilities, vitamin C controls collagen formation, a protein that gives your skin strength and elasticity. In other words, it helps your skin bounce back into shape instead of sag.

Multiple studies link a diet rich in vitamin C to better skin appearance. Fewer wrinkles and less dryness? Yes, please.

Remember, a single guava gives you twice the amount of vitamin C you need daily. More yummy fruit, younger-looking skin. It's a win-win.

Amazing source of lifesaving lycopene

Guava may be the number one raw source of lycopene, but — surprise — you can get three times the amount from another food — tomato juice.

How is this possible? It's pure science. Processing or cooking tomatoes breaks down their cell walls, making the lycopene in them more available to your body.

For instance, a cup of raw tomatoes has only 4.6 milligrams (mg) of lycopene. A cup of tomato juice rings in at a whopping 22 mg.

So fill your grocery buggy with products like tomato paste, tomato sauce, stewed tomatoes, and even ketchup, for a cartload of lycopene.

Want to get even more? Add olive oil to your recipe. The healthy fat increases antioxidant absorption.

Guava ingredients beat the blues

"To get rid of depression, I swim with dolphins," says TV personality Patti Stanger. That's great if you're retired in Florida, but what if you need a mood booster a little closer to home? Take a bite of nature's candy and you, too, may start feeling better.

That's right. Fruit is a natural blues blaster. "Women who ate at least two servings of fruit a day were less likely to suffer from depression than women who ate fewer servings," says Gita Mishra, professor at The University of Queensland School of Public Health in Australia. "We also found that eating two or more servings of fruit a day protected women from developing depression in the future."

While you should eat a variety of fruit to take advantage of all the vitamins and minerals they offer, here's what guava brings to the table — three depression-fighting nutrients.

Lycopene. Researchers found the more carotenoids in general you have in your system, the lower your chances of experiencing depression. And experts say lycopene is the most powerful carotenoid antioxidant. It was linked to fewer symptoms of depression in a Japanese study of close to 1,000 people. With levels around 8.6 milligrams (mg) a cup, guava is loaded with lycopene.

> Gaga for guava? You probably know you can buy different varieties. What you may not realize is redder guavas contain more lycopene. On the other hand, white guavas have more vitamin C. Get the best of both worlds and try 'em all.

Folate. A shortage of folate is considered a risk factor for severe depression, which is why some scientists think it may play a role in prevention. A cup of guava contains 20 percent of your daily folate.

Vitamin C. Dips in levels of this antioxidant are related to rocketing depression symptoms, according to a study of more than 300 folks age 65 and older. Scientists say that by easing damage to your cells, vitamin C may actually lessen anxiety. Get a whopping 600 percent of the C you need each day from just one cup of guava.

Guava leaf tea — a tasty way to balance blood sugar

Can guava help balance your blood sugar? Sure thing. Just brew up a nice cup of guava leaf tea. Plus, studies show it may even prevent type 2 diabetes.

You may not be familiar with guava leaf tea, but the beverage is big in Japan. It's no surprise then that Japanese researchers did a scientific review of everything they knew about guava leaf and glucose. They published these results in the journal *Nutrition & Metabolism*.

Take in a teacup to block sugar spikes. Whether you have diabetes, prediabetes, or you're just being cautious, a cup of guava tea with your meals may help ease your mind. The leaves can stop your body from absorbing certain sugars. That means your blood glucose levels don't shoot through the roof after you eat.

Keep sipping to steady sugar for the long haul. Check out this small study of men with prediabetes and mild type 2 diabetes. They drank guava leaf tea with every meal for 12 weeks, and all saw the same result — insulin and blood sugar levels dropped.

Some people think guava leaf tea tastes great on its own while others prefer to add a natural sweetener. Try it for yourself. You can find it online, in health food shops, or specialty markets.

Hempseed

2 reasons your heart loves hemp

Hempseed comes from a good plant with a bad reputation —
industrial hemp. It was once an American staple crop, used to
make items like cloth, paper, and rope. And now studies show
the seeds may help your heart.

Hold it right there — hemp? As in marijuana?

Nope.

Hempseed sold in the U.S. comes from the hemp plant — a
cousin of the marijuana plant — and has virtually no THC, the
active compound in marijuana. And as industry expert Chris
Conrad points out, "The cannabinoids are found, not in the
seeds, but in a completely separate part of the plant."

That means you can enjoy hempseed in its many forms —
seeds, oil, butter, and more — without worry.

Pack your diet with PUFAs for a happier heart. Because your
body can't make them, everyone needs to eat foods rich in
healthy fats, like polyunsaturated fatty acids (PUFAs).
Amazingly, hempseed contains significant amounts of both
omega-6 and omega-3 fatty acids, two PUFAs which lower cholesterol and blood pressure while fighting inflammation.

And in hempseed, these fatty acids are present in an almost-perfect
ratio, which is rather rare and extremely important to good health.

Even though hempseed has not been a booming topic for researchers, a study published in the *European Journal of Nutrition* showed two tablespoons of hempseed oil a day for four weeks lowered total-to-HDL cholesterol ratio better than flaxseed oil, a proven heart-healthy food.

Slash your risk of heart disease with amino acids. Your body also can't make amino acids, the building blocks of protein. That's OK because you can get them from wholesome foods like hempseed.

In fact, hempseed oil contains surprisingly high levels of a particular amino acid, arginine. It plays a role in producing nitric oxide, a molecule that helps balance blood pressure, support healthy blood vessels, and control blood clots and inflammation.

A study of more than 13,000 people revealed you may be able to lower your risk of heart disease by choosing more arginine-rich foods.

Slip hemp into your diet with 4 tasty treats

People are hooked on the nutty flavor of hempseed. If you want to give it a go, you're in luck. Hempseed products are gaining ground and now come in all shapes and sizes, from hemp butter, flour, cheese, and coffee to powdered hemp protein. Check out the most popular hempseed products on the market and learn how to add them to your diet.

Whole hempseed. Whole seeds retain their crunchy outer shell, which means they offer more insoluble fiber, but make it harder for your body to digest the seed's protein.

Hemp hearts. The most common hemp product at the supermarket is the soft inner seed. Look for labels that say hemp hearts, hulled or shelled hempseed, or even hemp nuts. Sprinkle onto salads and yogurt or bake into muffins.

Hempseed oil. Wherever you need an oil in a low-heat recipe, this is a delicious alternative. Experts especially recommend it for cold recipes because high temps can destroy the health benefits. Drizzle it on salads, steamed veggies, or rice.

Hempseed milk. A glass of this milk is rich in omega-3 and omega-6 fatty acids and, if unsweetened, has fewer calories than 1 percent milk. As for the taste, many people describe it as earthy.

You can get hemp products in stores or online, but like many specialty products, they can be pricey. For the longest shelf life and best nutrition, keep hempseeds and oil in your freezer or fridge.

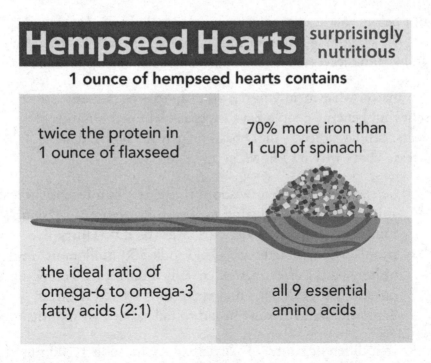

Hempseed Hearts — surprisingly nutritious

1 ounce of hempseed hearts contains

twice the protein in 1 ounce of flaxseed

70% more iron than 1 cup of spinach

the ideal ratio of omega-6 to omega-3 fatty acids (2:1)

all 9 essential amino acids

Holy basil

Sip from the holy grail of stress-reducing herbs

"Reality is the leading cause of stress among those in touch with it," jokes actress Lily Tomlin. You can't get rid of every stressful situation in your life. But you can give your body the extra boost it needs to face hard times head-on — like a cup of holy basil tea. This relaxing herb has a long history of nipping stress symptoms in the bud.

But before you head to your spice cabinet, hold on. Holy basil is not the sweet basil found in your favorite pesto recipes. These fragrant, bitter leaves are more commonly found in teas or capsules.

No matter what form you try, you can expect the same stress-relieving benefits people have experienced for thousands of years. Studies agree — holy basil helps your body adapt to stress. That's why it's known as an adaptogen.

- Scientists put ancient wisdom to the test in a recent clinical study. Difficulty adjusting to stressful situations is a symptom of generalized anxiety disorder (GAD). Thirty-five people who suffered with GAD took 500 milligrams (mg) of holy basil leaf extract twice daily after meals. Follow-up questionnaires showed that symptoms related to stress, depression, and anxiety began to fade after two months.

- In a different study, 71 participants who took 1,200 mg of holy basil daily reported improvements for stress-related symptoms in just six weeks. That means less forgetfulness, exhaustion, and sleep difficulties. And as a bonus, no negative side effects. That's more than you can say for most anxiety medications.

Holy basil is still new to modern science, so researchers haven't recommended a dosage yet. But if you want to give it a try, you can buy tea online or in stores.

Many happy Amazon customers say holy basil helps them relax and even sleep better. And prices for this soothing tea are on par with other healthful teas.

3 types of holy basil you'll want to try

What's the easiest way to score holy basil benefits? Buy from health food stores or online in the form of dried leaves or supplements. But with a little creativity, you can use other types to help your health.

- Powder. Find this fine form in health stores or online. Use it to make tea, or sprinkle on vegetables

- Essential oil. Sellers say diffusing the warm aroma will help calm your mind and encourage sleep.

- Fresh leaves. It's hard to find fresh holy basil since it grows best in the climate of its native India. Try growing it indoors in a pot on a sunny windowsill.

Tulsi for tumors — an herb with incomparable benefits

Holy moley! Shop for holy basil, and you'll come across something strange — packages also labeled tulsi. That's because tulsi is another word for this heavenly herb. It translates to "incomparable one." A good name, considering its powerful effects against cancer.

So how is tulsi such a fierce cancer foe? Eugenol, apigenin, luteolin, and a few other words that seem impossible to pronounce. These seemingly nonsensical terms have one thing in common — they're all phytochemicals, natural compounds found in plants. Their superpower is tackling cancer and warding off damage from radiation therapy.

Holy basil sounds like an angelic herb. But if you're taking medications that thin blood, like heparin or warfarin — even aspirin — it can be downright devilish. Like those drugs, the herb slows clotting, so it may increase your chances of bruising and bleeding.

Antioxidants fight cancer footholds. Your body is made up of millions of cells. Cancer gains ground when damaged cells grow and spread. Phytochemicals in holy basil protect your body by acting like antioxidants. They squash dangerous cells, blocking the development of cancer.

As a result, this "saintly" herb may prevent an impressive lineup of cancers from hijacking your body. Basil bodyguards may help halt skin, liver, oral, prostate, and lung cancers.

Fight off treatment effects with ancient herb. Killing cancer cells with radiation is a common treatment. While high-dose radiation destroys cancer cells and shrinks tumors, it can also harm healthy cells in the process. This is why many people experience side effects such as nausea, skin irritation, fatigue, diarrhea, and more.

Studies show tulsi and its phytochemicals protect against the effects of radiation therapy. They scavenge free radicals to prevent radiation from damaging your healthy cells.

Although supplements are available, tulsi is still considered an alternative medicine. Scientists haven't performed enough studies to make a recommendation for cancer prevention. So talk to your doctor before adding tulsi supplements to your cancer-fighting arsenal.

Balance blood sugar with an ancient healer

Holy basil is a powerful herb in Indian medicine. For thousands of years, Ayurvedic medicine, as it's known, has prescribed it for a hodgepodge of complaints — pain, inflammation, skin conditions, colds, fevers, and more.

You won't find many Western studies on these alternative uses. But you can dig up an occasional diamond in the rough. Who would have thought holy basil could help fight a serious condition like diabetes? Yet research shows it may play a role in balancing blood sugar.

Researchers first studied this herb back in the 1960s. They found holy basil improved fasting blood sugar in nine out of 10 people with type 2 diabetes. Fast forward three decades. Researchers asked type 2 diabetes patients to take 2.5 grams — a little more than a tablespoon — of tulsi leaves every day for a month.

Again, blood sugar levels improved. After an eight-hour fast, volunteers' blood glucose dropped about 18 percent. Post-meal glucose levels improved by more than 7 percent. Recent studies have continued to support holy basil as a safe treatment that may help normalize blood sugar.

In India, holy basil is still more commonly used in folk medicine rather than culinary dishes. But countries such as Thailand take advantage of its spicy taste in their cooking. Follow their lead and toss it into stir-fries and soups.

Kale

This queen of greens eases arthritis woes

Another birthday sails by, and you feel as burned out as those candles on your cake. Painful, stiff joints are making it hard to enjoy life. Just a natural part of getting older, right? Not necessarily. All hail kale, the queen of greens. Just one-third cup of this veggie superfood every day can help ease your joint stiffness, protect your cartilage, and cut your arthritis pain.

This salad bar superstar dishes up healthier joints. Studies show kale's nutrients protect your joints and slow down cartilage damage. Scientists think it's the veggie's compound, sulforaphane, that blocks the enzymes and molecules responsible for joint damage and inflammation. And that means less pain and stiffness for you.

Chewing a bite of raw kale — or chopping the leaves on your cutting board — gets this sulforaphane churning. The chewing or chopping action causes kale's enzyme, myrosinase, to activate. When it combines with other kale compounds, sulforaphane is created. It's sort of like snapping a glow stick to mix the chemicals that make the light come on.

But wait. If you're going to cook your kale, unless you use a certain "chop and stop" trick, you may destroy all that healthy sulforaphane before it has a chance to form. Simply chop your kale, and then set your timer for 40 minutes before exposing it to heat. When time is up, the sulforaphane is ready to go.

Are you using frozen kale? "Chop and stop" won't work. Frozen vegetables are flash-cooked before freezing, and this process destroys the myrosinase. No myrosinase, no sulforaphane.

But there is a fix. Mustard greens are also cruciferous veggies, so their seeds contain the enzymes needed to make the sulforaphane. Pick up some ground mustard seed, available in the spice aisle at your grocery store, and sprinkle it on your cooked kale. Just a pinch will do the trick.

Collagen, cartilage, and vitamin C. Osteoarthritis destroys your cartilage, leaving you with painful, swollen joints. But kale can help put a stop to all that. The green veggie is rich in vitamin C, just what your body needs to make collagen — an important building block for cartilage.

Vitamin C can also protect you from the cartilage-crushing free radicals floating around in your system. Researchers think these free radicals — molecules that can damage your cells and DNA — might also break down your cartilage. Antioxidants like vitamin C stop free radicals in their tracks.

Kale and its cousins, a vitamin-packed bunch that includes broccoli, cabbage, and rutabagas, are all part of the *Brassicaceae* plant family. The group's alternate name is *Cruciferae*, a Latin word referring to the four petals that grow in the form of a crucifix or cross-like shape in the plants' flowers. And that's where the term "cruciferous" comes from.

Adding just a third of a cup of vitamin-rich kale to your diet every day is a great way to start. Want a little more? A delicious cup of raw kale gives you 134 percent of your daily recommended amount of vitamin C.

Feast your eyes on kale

Faster than a speeding bullet. More powerful than a locomotive. Sure, he could leap tall buildings with a single bound. But best of all? Superman had super sight. Makes you wonder if the citizens of Krypton knew about kale's eye-popping powers. This leafy green can't guarantee you'll have Superman's X-ray vision, but it does contain compounds that can wage war against a modern enemy of your eyes — blue light.

There's a rainbow connection. Red, orange, yellow, green, blue, indigo, violet. ROYGBIV from science class. A simple way to remember the colors of the visible light spectrum in order from the longest wavelength to the shortest — the way they're arranged in a rainbow. Blue, the color with one of the shortest wavelengths, produces a high amount of energy. So it has the potential to do a lot of damage to your eyes.

Many of the light sources you're exposed to today — including digital screens like computers and smartphones, fluorescent lighting, and even the sun — contain a significant amount of blue light. Bet you didn't know light-emitting diode (LED) bulbs put off more blue light than traditional incandescent bulbs.

Blue light has a dark side. Why is blue light bad for you? Because it reaches deep into your eyes where it can cause damage to the retina, leading to everything from poor vision to age-related macular degeneration (AMD).

And a recent study at the University of Houston found blue light can interfere with your sleep. When blue light was blocked for three hours before bedtime, people showed a 58-percent increase in melatonin levels, the chemical that tells your system it's time to sleep. Less blue light, better shuteye.

Block the blues with greens. Two of kale's antioxidants, lutein and zeaxanthin, keep your peepers safe from dangerous blue light. Sort of like eye spies, these two compounds hide out in your retina's macular pigment, in just the right spot to soak up harmful blue light wavelengths before they reach the light-sensitive cells deep in your eyes.

Your body can't make its own lutein and zeaxanthin, though, so it's up to you to get the amount experts consider most beneficial — 10 milligrams (mg) of lutein and 2 mg of zeaxanthin every day. It's not hard. One cup of chopped, raw kale provides more than 26 mg of lutein and zeaxanthin combined.

So pile that kale on your plate, and who knows? Maybe X-ray vision, and a better night's sleep, can be yours. Quick as a wink.

Too much of a good thing?

Vitamin K helps your blood clot. That's one of its main jobs. And cruciferous veggies like kale are jam-packed with it. In fact, one cup of chopped raw kale contains 547 micrograms of vitamin K. Now that may not seem like a whole lot, but those meager micrograms add up to around five times your daily recommended amount.

So is this too much of a good thing? If you're taking blood thinners like warfarin (Coumadin), then the answer is yes. Warfarin's job is to stop your blood from clotting. Too much vitamin K can work against it.

Unless your doctor says so, you don't have to avoid vitamin K-rich foods. Just keep your intake steady, so your medication works the way it's supposed to.

Keep your memories crystal clear

Corn has it. Squash has it. Even broccoli and grapes have it. What is it? Lutein, an antioxidant that can slow down — or even prevent — age-related memory problems. But do you know which food has the most? You guessed it — kale.

Researchers say people who have more lutein in their blood also have more gray matter in their brain. Well, at least in their parahippocampal cortex, the part of the brain that plays a role in preserving — wait for it — your crystallized intelligence.

Bet you didn't even know you had one of those, but it's the term for your ability to hold onto the skills, knowledge, and experience it's taken you a lifetime to build up. You don't want to lose all that, and kale's lutein is there to help.

Scientists recently studied nearly 80 seniors to learn about the relationship between lutein, crystallized intelligence, and the brain's gray matter. Their tests confirmed lutein is linked to crystallized intelligence and may slow or even block memory loss by putting the brakes on brain aging.

Scientists aren't sure exactly how the lutein works, though. It may be through its role as an anti-inflammatory, or it might help with cell-to-cell signaling — an important process that allows cells to grow and work normally.

So how much lutein do you need? Although there is no recommended amount, experts suggest a healthy daily supplement would contain about 10 milligrams. But you can get yours straight from the garden. One cup of cooked kale contains double that. So go ahead. Help yourself to a little food for thought.

Kale tales: how to pick and prepare this keen green

There they are. The bundles of colorful kale arranged on your market's produce shelves. You'd like to give the leafy greens a try, but how do you know what kind to choose? And what about all the prepping and cooking?

You may think it's easier to steer your cart off in a different direction, in search of a safer, more garden-variety choice of greens. Like old reliable iceberg lettuce, perhaps. But don't miss out on all the goodness kale has to offer. Instead, use these tips to pick and fix the kind of kale that's just right for you.

> Searching for a way to get the antioxidant goodness of brassica veggies — without kale's bitter taste? Enjoy a cup of tea. Broccoli tea, that is. Just one cup provides 15 milligrams of glucoraphanin, the substance your body turns into arthritis-fighting sulforaphane. And — surprise! — there's no broccoli taste. Look for broccoli teas and coffees online.

At the store. These are the three most common types of kale, the ones you're likely see at your supermarket.

- Curly kale is the most popular variety. It has tight, ruffled leaves, usually in different shades of green, but sometimes you'll even see purple. Its peppery flavor can be very bitter, but it's the most versatile — and the most forgiving of first-time kale cooks.

- Lacinato kale, nicknamed dinosaur kale, has a scaly texture and a dark bluish-green color. Not as bitter as curly kale, this type has flat leaves that hold on to their texture even after cooking. A great choice for making kale chips.

- Red Russian kale resembles little oak leaves. Its purple stalks are usually discarded because their texture makes them hard to chew. But the leaves are sweeter and have a more delicate flavor than other varieties.

In the kitchen. Kale tends to get more bitter the longer you store it, so it's best to eat it within two or three days. To prepare, thoroughly wash the vegetable under cold water, using your fingers to rub both sides of the leaves. Next, tenderize your kale with these easy tips.

- Cut out the large center stems, and then massage the leaves with your hands. This starts the breakdown of cellulose, which makes the leaves less tough and releases the nutrients.

- Recipe calls for lots of kale? Place a few cups of the raw chopped veggie in a plastic zipper-lock bag that's been left slightly open. Push down on the bag with your rolling pin for two to three minutes.

- Try this chef's trick for extra-tender cooked kale. Wash the cut leaves thoroughly and sprinkle them with baking soda or baking powder before cooking.

After chopping, remember to wait 40 minutes before you cook to allow kale's healthy compound — sulforaphane — to form. And blanch kale first if you plan to sauté it right away, or if you want to freeze the greens to use later. Stir the fresh kale into boiling water for one or two minutes. Drain and run under cold water immediately.

Kiwi

A super source of 'C' restores body and brain

"Someone once threw me a small, brown, hairy kiwi fruit, and I threw a wastebasket over it until it was dead," joked journalist Erma Bombeck. You may have had the same reaction upon seeing a kiwi for the first time. They aren't the prettiest fruits on the outside. But on the inside, kiwi is a powerhouse of vitamin C and other nutrients that just might transform your health.

Veto viruses with a vital nutrient. Feel something coming on? The time-honored advice is to get more C, the mighty vitamin famous for immune system support. It may even help you fight upper respiratory tract infections. This is a big deal as you age, because symptoms like congestion, cough, and sore throat can quickly turn into something more dangerous.

In addition to almost one-and-a-half times the amount of vitamin C you need each day for good health, kiwis contain vitamin E, folate, polyphenols, and carotenoids — all of which help support your immune system and fight infection.

Scientists put this fun fruit to the test. They asked seniors to eat either four gold kiwis or two bananas every day for a month. Those with head congestion and sore throats felt better faster if they were in the kiwi group.

Toss back two fruits to soothe your state of mind. There's only one thing that can bring you down faster than a virus, and that's a bad mood. Turns out, vitamin C may regulate brain chemicals that affect how you feel.

And other nutrients found in kiwis — B vitamins, vitamins E and K, and carotenoids — also contribute to a better disposition.

For six weeks, 35 young men ate either one-half a gold kiwi or two of the fuzzy fruits every day. Those lucky enough to be placed in the two-kiwi group were able to tone down some of those telltale signs of a bad mood, including anger and anxiety. Plus, they experienced a 32-percent drop in depression and a bump in energy.

Pause on pills: supplements can't replace a healthy diet

Sure, popping a multivitamin or downing a handful of supplements is a fast and easy way to get certain nutrients. But don't think that's a smart substitute for nourishing foods, like the kiwi. Studies say multivitamins and supplements are not all they're cracked up to be and may even be harmful. Vitamin C, vitamin E, and beta carotene — all members of the kiwi crew and necessary for good health — are some of the stars of these studies.

The problem with choosing pills over whole foods, experts warn, is they may not actually reduce your risk for health concerns or prolong your life. In fact, megadoses of vitamins and minerals could be harmful, ballooning your chances of heart failure and cancer.

Stick to the real deal — whole foods. And talk to your doctor before you waste your money on pointless pills.

Fuzzy fruit gets to the heart of ticker troubles

Looking for a fresh way to fortify your heart? How about a juicy Chinese gooseberry.

Your "no way" might turn into a resounding "yes" when you learn this is really just another name for the beloved kiwi fruit. The Chinese gooseberry may have been renamed by the New Zealand agricultural industry to sound more appealing, but the heart benefits have always been close at hand.

Chalk it up to vitamin C and polyphenols that act as antioxidants, say scientists. Kiwi is packed with them. And they may be the reason the tasty fruit protects against heart disease and stroke. Antioxidants defend your heart and blood vessels against damaging free radicals.

Beat the two villains of heart hiccups. By far, the biggest threats to heart health are high blood pressure and high cholesterol. Both skyrocket your risk for heart disease by pressuring your ticker to work harder. Scientists agree kiwis help combat this duo.

- Blood pressure. More than 100 people with high BP ate either three kiwi fruits or one apple a day for eight weeks. Those eating kiwis came away with lower blood pressure.

- Cholesterol. Out of more than 1,400 folks, those who ate at least one kiwi each week had higher HDL "good" cholesterol levels and lower amounts of fat in their blood than those who ate less.

Slash stroke risk with just one kiwi a week. When blood flow to an area of the brain is cut off, a stroke strikes. The most common cause is a blood clot. But kiwis have a secret weapon for your veins, according to a Spanish study published in *Nutrition Journal.*

Those who ate at least one kiwi every week had lower fibrinogen levels than those who did not snack on the fruit this regularly. Fibrinogen is a protein that helps your blood clot. If you have high amounts, you also have a higher risk of heart-related issues like stroke and blood vessel blockages to other parts of your body.

2 quick tricks to serve up kiwi

Kiwi skins are completely edible — and even offer added fiber. But if you're just not into woolly brown peels, here are two nifty ways to eat a kiwi without its skin.

- Quick peel. Cut off both ends. Run a spoon along the inside of the peel to remove the inner fruit.

- Fruit cups. Cut the kiwi in half. You'll be left with two mini-cups. Just scoop out the goods with your spoon.

Avoid tummy upsets — eat this for dessert

Feeling bloated or backed up? Dessert may be the answer.

Sure, sweet treats don't sound like a cure for constipation. But choose kiwi after a meal, and you may get the relief you've been searching for.

Whether in a smoothie, sorbet, or tart, or part of a simple salad, squeeze two or three kiwis into your day for a few weeks. You'll find trips to the bathroom are more frequent and less painful. And you'll feel better in between. Here's why.

- Fiber. Want to give your bowels the green light? Fiber is the ultimate traffic control. It softens and enlarges stools to keep things moving along. Your best bet — green kiwi. It has a bit more fiber than the gold variety.

- Actinidin. This enzyme in kiwis breaks down proteins in food, especially those found in favorites such as yogurt, cheese, and fish. Some experts think it also stimulates receptors in your colon to encourage movement. What a yummy way to break up a traffic jam.

Hit the sack with this bedtime snack

Without doubt, kiwis are great for a host of health problems. But when's the best time to eat them? If you struggle with sleeplessness, graze an hour before bedtime.

That's what scientists suggested after winding up a small study on kiwis and sleep patterns. They recruited people with sleep problems and had them eat two kiwis one hour before bedtime. After a month, they reported going to sleep faster and staying asleep longer.

Researchers say antioxidants such as flavonoids, antho-cyanins, and carotenoids are responsible. In addition, kiwi's serotonin and folate can help you get the shuteye you need without the sheep.

For a twist on this classic treat, go for the gold. Gold kiwis are a little harder to find than green, but worth the effort. They have more vitamin C, fewer seeds, and a thinner, smoother skin.

Lactobacillus

Forget eating an apple a day — good germs keep the doctor away

Bacteria are enemies to your health and home. That's what you've always been told, right? So you wipe down your kitchen counters with bleach and scrub your hands with antibacterial soap, hoping you'll fend off food poisoning, infections, and deadly diseases.

But all bacteria aren't bad news. Your body is home to trillions of friendly bacteria that help you digest food, metabolize medicine, and fight off harmful germs.

This community is called your microbiome. It contains hundreds of different species of bacteria — both good and bad. Usually the good guys keep the disease-causing germs in check, but sometimes the balance shifts. And if bad bacteria have the upper hand, you'll get sick.

Be proactive to tip the balance back towards good bacteria. Live cultures of helpful bacteria, called probiotics, give your immune system an extra push. Researchers studied hundreds of different bacteria and found *lactobacillus* is your best bet for fending off harmful germs.

Lactobacillus can refer to dozens of different species of bacteria from the same genus, with one important thing in common.

They produce lactic acid when they digest sugars, which helps kill disease-causing bacteria lurking in your gut.

As unappetizing as it may sound, you'll find these bacteria in many of your favorite foods. Cheese, yogurt, naturally fermented pickles, and even sourdough bread all get their tangy flavors from the lactic acid these bacteria create.

Feel a cold coming on? Liven up your diet. If you want to harness all the health benefits of *lactobacillus*, start eating foods loaded with live bacteria. According to a Finnish study, cheese containing live cultures of *lactobacillus* can fight age-related changes in your immune system.

Researchers fed a group of healthy, elderly people a slice of plain cheese with breakfast for two weeks. After that, they spent four weeks eating a probiotic cheese loaded with more than a billion colony-forming units (CFUs) of *lactobacillus* bacteria. Then they ate the control cheese again for four more weeks.

The scientists measured the older people's immune systems throughout the study and found their natural defenses increased while eating the probiotic cheese.

> The older you get, the more trouble your immune system has responding to threats. That leaves your aging body open to infection, chronic inflammation, autoimmune disorders, even cancer. Probiotics are an easy way to power up your immune system.

Another study may have an explanation for the probiotic's success. It found that *lactobacillus* stimulates large white blood cells called macrophages to respond to inflammation. This quick response helps your immune system fight off dangerous threats.

Scan the labels of yogurt, cheese, or other specialty foods to check for immune-boosting probiotics, especially *lactobacillus*. And if you can't find one you like, supplements are an option, too.

Tame tummy troubles with a little help from your friends

The bacteria in your gut outnumber the stars in the night sky. Your digestive tract is home to more than 100 trillion micro-organisms working to keep it in tiptop shape. But sometimes you need to reboot your microbiome, and nothing works better than *lactobacillus*. Here are three ways these friendly bacteria can overhaul your digestion.

Good bacteria lead the crackdown on Crohn's and colitis. Inflammatory bowel disease (IBD) refers to two different conditions — ulcerative colitis (UC) and Crohn's disease (CD). Both these diseases cause painful, chronic inflammation in your intestines. Scientists aren't quite sure what triggers this disease, but your immune system might be to blame. When your body tries to fend off invading viruses or bacteria, your own intestines get caught in the fray.

According to a recent review of 27 studies, *lactobacillus* supplements could soothe the diarrhea, cramping, and pain associated with IBD. They work by creating a shield for your intestines, preventing harmful bacteria and your immune system from triggering inflammation.

Keep your gut in check to manage irritable bowel syndrome. Cramping, bloating, gas, diarrhea, and constipation aren't easy to talk about. But if you suffer from irritable bowel syndrome (IBS), the pain and discomfort is always on your mind.

A little *lactobacillus* will help you fight this chronic condition. Researchers think IBS may be caused by an unhealthy amount of bad bacteria in your system, so you need to focus on balancing your microbiome to get your digestion back on track.

Early studies suggest *lactobacillus* supplements can re-establish healthy bacterial colonies in your gut. Scientists have had success with a variety of different species, but everybody's gut is different. Try a few different probiotics to see what works for you.

Two ways to outrun the runs. Believe it or not, diarrhea clocks in at number two among the most reported illnesses in the United States. This common condition could be caused by anything that shakes up your gastro system, like a bad burrito, a virus, or even your medicine. If you're suffering from certain kinds of chronic diarrhea, *lactobacillus* can put your digestion back on track.

- Antibiotic-associated diarrhea. One out of every five people taking antibiotics comes down with a nasty case of diarrhea. That's because antibiotics kill bacteria — good and bad. So sometimes your prescription drugs take out the microbes in charge of keeping your gut healthy.

  Usually this problem clears up by itself, but probiotics can give you a little extra help. Evidence suggests *lactobacillus* supplements could help manage diarrhea associated with antibiotic use. Just be sure to talk to your doctor before trying this out. And don't stop taking your antibiotics without consulting him first.

- Radiation therapy is a double-edged sword. It kills deadly cancer cells, but this treatment often kills healthy cells, too. If the lining of your intestines get damaged, you'll suffer from severe bouts of diarrhea. Fortunately, *lactobacillus* helps you fight back. Studies reveal supplements loaded with these friendly bacteria can help relieve diarrhea symptoms.

Don't let your gut feelings get you down

People think with their stomachs — literally. Your microbiome lives in your gut, but it controls more than just digestion. These trillions of bacteria play a role in issues you may think start in your head, like anxiety, stress, and depression.

Researchers have long thought probiotic supplements can help ease depression and anxiety, but a new study published in the *Journal of Affective Disorders* finally confirmed their suspicions. People with major depressive disorder have lower than normal levels of *lactobacillus* in their gut. So getting a dose of these friendly bacteria might help you ward off the blues.

In one study, a group of healthy people took either a beverage fermented with *L. casei* or a placebo. After three weeks, people who used probiotics improved their mood more than those using the placebo. Even better, people who showed early signs of depression boosted their moods the most.

One way researchers thought *lactobacillus* helped was by treating a major physical trigger of stress — poor digestion. But people's moods improved regardless of their gut health.

It turns out *lactobacillus* may actually change the way your brain works. Animal studies conducted by Canadian researchers found *L. rhamnosus* helps maintain healthy levels of a neurotransmitter called gamma-aminobutyric acid (GABA). This chemical sends signals to your brain to help keep everything in balance.

Feeling anxious, stressed, or depressed? Your GABA levels could be out of whack. Try eating more foods with *lactobacillus*, especially *L. casei* or *L. rhamnosus*, the strains shown to boost mood.

4 trusty rules for probiotic shopping

Probiotics come in everything from yogurt to pickles, but how do you really know what you're getting? Follow these rules and you'll be a probiotic pro in no time.

Get on a first-name basis. The first things you need to know about a probiotic are its genus, species, and strain. Reputable products should give the entire name, like *Lactobacillus acidophilus NCFM*.

Play the numbers game. Look for the colony-forming units (CFUs) to know how many live bacteria the product has.

Keep it fresh. Check dates to make sure you're not paying for bacteria that died months ago. And check to make sure it's been stored properly, too. Most probiotics last longer at cool temperatures.

Don't get duped. Independent tests showed five out of 19 supplements didn't have all the advertised bacteria. Look for certified supplements or products with the "Live and Active Cultures" seal.

Work from the inside out to trim your waistline

Diet and exercise are supposed to tip the scales in your favor, but sometimes weeks of hard work barely move the needle. If that's the case, it's time to focus on your gut — specifically, the trillions of bacteria living inside of it.

Experts think the gut bacteria of obese people create too many short-chain fatty acids (SCFAs) when they eat carbohydrates. In turn, these SCFAs slow down your digestion, causing you to absorb more nutrients — and fat — that can pack on the pounds. Want to fight back? Try kick-starting your weight loss with a dose of friendly bacteria.

Lactobacillus for the win. In a recent study, overweight women and men took either a placebo or two capsules loaded with 160 million colony-forming units (CFUs) of *L. rhamnosus* every day. After just three months, the women taking the probiotic lost almost 10 pounds on average, compared to just 6 pounds on the placebo.

Even better, probiotic losers continued to lose weight. Researchers checked in after another 12 weeks and found the women who used *L. rhamnosus* lost almost 2 more pounds. But the weight of those who took the placebo stayed the same.

L. rhamnosus actually lowered the levels of gut bacteria related to obesity. And as an added bonus, it caused a drop in the hormone that helps control your appetite.

Give your gut a variety. Unfortunately, the probiotic did not affect weight loss in the men who participated. Researchers aren't sure why, but sometimes people react better to different species of *lactobacillus*. A recent review found evidence that *L. gasseri* and *L. amylovorus* are also good choices for people trying to lose weight.

Just remember, as helpful as probiotics may be, they can't do it all. If you want to get the most out of them, researchers say you should also eat a diet low in fat and high in fiber.

Legumes

Beans 'n things — snag health perks with protein-packed grub

"Some people think the plant-based, whole foods diet is extreme," says Dr. Caldwell Esselstyn Jr. in the documentary *Forks Over Knives*. "Half a million people a year will have their chests opened up and a vein taken from their leg and sewn onto their coronary artery. Some people would call that extreme."

Sure, chowing down on fruits and veggies full-time can be a big adjustment. But with so many tasty options and health bonuses — like a lower risk of heart disease, cancer, obesity, and cataracts — you may come to find clean eating isn't such a sacrifice after all.

In fact, lay a foundation of lip-smacking legumes, and this way of eating could be a gateway to a whole new you.

Fabulous fare starts with a helping of legumes. Beans, peas, peanuts, and lentils — legumes come in all tastes and sizes. And their powerful nutrients make them a yummy transition to healthy plant-based or vegetarian diets.

A forkful of legumes is packed with protein, fiber, and vitamins and minerals like folate and iron. But to get the most out of these delicious dishes, experts say to aim for at least three servings a day. A serving includes:

- a quarter cup of bean dip or hummus.

- half cup of lentils, split peas, cooked beans, tofu, or tempeh.

- full cup of peas or sprouted lentils.

Pull a scrumptious switcheroo to add years to your life.
"Where do you get your protein?" It's the question vegetarians grow tired of hearing. Why? Meat isn't the only food filled with this necessary nutrient. Plant foods are also packed with protein.

A cup of white beans has 17.4 grams of protein, compared to a hamburger patty's 19.8 grams. Not bad for a bowl of beans.

> Beans, beans, they're good for your health, the darker they are, the more they help. Why are colored beans so superb? They have two to three times more antioxidant power than white beans, according to one study. What a great reason to pick up more red, navy, and black varieties.

But here's the kicker. Studies show a link between red meat and conditions like heart disease. Wholesome plant choices, on the other hand, have no downside. That's why many experts recommend a shift from animal to plant protein.

To drive the point home, a recent study put the two types of protein to the test. They collected data from more than 130,000 participants and published the results in *JAMA Internal Medicine*. Their conclusion? A simple switch to plant protein could lower your chances of an early death.

Even if vegetarianism doesn't work for you, a transition to a more plant-based diet is pretty easy. Restrict meat to just once or twice a week, and sub in legumes. You'll lower your risk for health hurdles like high blood sugar, blood pressure, and cho-lesterol. Plus, you may see a disappearing act on that excess belly fat. Cool beans.

Defy the deadly quartet with a special sort of legume

In the midst of unhealthy lifestyle choices lies the deadly quartet — an army of abdominal obesity, high blood sugar, high triglycerides, and high blood pressure.

Stick to bad food and exercise habits, and you could be fighting a losing battle against these four conditions known as metabolic syndrome. But take legumes for a taste test and you'll lower your chances of developing heart disease, diabetes, and stroke.

Don't eat just any legume though. You want pulses, the kind that come dried like peas and beans. With this delicious all-purpose health food, you can eat cheap and still eat well. Add these top 10 healthy foods to your table, all for under $1 per cup — lentils, chickpeas, peas, kidney beans, cannellini beans, navy beans, fava beans, black beans, pinto beans, and black-eyed peas.

Shrink a tubby tummy with fabulous fiber. Abdominal fat, the kind that gathers around your organs, increases your risk for disease and death. But pulses can help banish belly fat in more ways than one.

First, they make you feel fuller after a meal — particularly com-pared to meat — which can control your hunger for hours and hours. Then, they help you eat less during your next meal. This can help you not only drop the pounds, but also lower body fat, says a recent study published in *The American Journal of Clinical Nutrition.*

Experts say you owe it to the fiber. A cup of chickpeas contains half of the fiber you need each day.

"Simply including pulses in your diet may help you lose weight, and we think more importantly, prevent you from gaining it back after you lose it," says lead author Dr. Russell de Souza.

Steadfast pair balances sugar surges. Every person with diabetes should be eating legumes. Why? Dozens of trials show that chowing down on pulses can help control diabetes. They lower sugar spikes and insulin resistance. And chickpeas may be the best.

Maybe it's the fiber. Or perhaps it's the resistant starch, which like fiber, doesn't break down in your stomach. Both slow down absorption to fend off sugar rushes and feed good gut bacteria. These bacteria help nurture your immune system and steady your sugar levels.

A few a day keeps your arteries open for business. Heart-healthy pulses can demolish "bad" cholesterol, lowering your risk of heart disease.

In one study, adding two daily servings of lentils, chickpeas, beans, or split peas slashed cholesterol levels. For many participants, numbers even dropped below the range that calls for statin drugs.

The magic, once again, is in the fiber. Pulses contain whopping amounts of soluble and insoluble fiber. Both keep your body from absorbing lipids like cholesterol and triglycerides. This naturally leads to lower levels of artery-clogging fats in your blood.

Haul down high BP to heal your heart. Folks without legumes in their daily diet may have four times the risk of getting high blood pressure.

Pulses are high in fiber, protein, and potassium. All of these nutrients are a boon to your blood pressure. Lower BP eases the pressure on your ticker, which equals a healthier heart.

Many studies use one to two servings of legumes daily. That's a half to one cup of cooked beans each day — an easy, and tasty, way to a balanced body.

Easy as pie — beans fill in for pricey bakeware

Does your dessert recipe call for blind baking? Relax. You don't have to use a blindfold. This method simply means pre-baking your crust before you add the filling. To keep the dough from bubbling up in the oven, you can buy fancy ceramic pie weights. Or save your cash, and use dried beans.

If you make a fruit tart, for example, you don't want to ruin the treat by baking the filling. This calls for a blind bake.

Put a layer of parchment paper or foil on the pie crust, and fill with dried beans. Halfway through cooking, remove the makeshift pie weight to let the bottom of the pie shell cook all the way through.

The beans will get extra dry, so you won't want to eat them after. But you can keep them to reuse next time.

Amp up your aging body lentil by lentil

"You can't help getting older, but you don't have to get old," said George Burns who continued to work in the entertainment industry until his death at age 100. How do you keep your body young? A legume-loaded diet is a good start. Beans, peas, and lentils are packed with a pair of nutrients that fight off two major agers — muscle and bone loss.

Bulk up with powerful protein. If you're 75 or older, you've probably heard of sarcopenia. It's a condition connected to old age and loss of muscle strength and function. Picture losing your balance often or being unable to complete everyday tasks, like lifting groceries.

Physical activity is the number one way to combat muscle loss. But for all-over support, add some legumes to your strategy. Spooning an extra helping of beans on your plate delivers a punch of protein. The average Joe needs about 50 grams of protein each day. A cup of lentils provides 36 percent of the recommendation.

Proteins are made of amino acids. And legumes contain a special one called leucine. Leucine plays an important role in powering up muscles. That's why experts encourage older folks to eat a diet high in essential amino acids, particularly leucine-rich foods such as legumes.

Build up bones the antioxidant way. Seniority comes with outward signs like wrinkles. But sometimes the biggest markers of aging are ones you can't see. Bone loss, known as osteopenia, is a silent hazard. But a unique antioxidant in legumes — phytate — may help fight bone loss.

People who eat more high-phytate foods may have stronger bones, says a study published in the *Journal of Medicinal Food*. Brawny bones serve up a lower risk of major fracture, particularly broken hips.

In another study, researchers measured phytate levels in a group of 157 postmenopausal women. They found that ladies with the highest phytate levels had the lowest levels of bone loss in their spine and hip.

How do beans do it? Experts think phytates may protect against bone loss by making sure healthy bones don't break down. Think of them as your 24-hour support team.

3 powerful nutrients crush cancer

Experts recently spilled the beans on legumes. They say bean nutrients take a stand against certain cancers, including colon, breast, and prostate cancer. Here's how.

Flavonoids stop cancer cells from traveling. Plant compounds called flavonoids could be behind the tumor-fighting powers of legumes. They're a triple threat against cancer, particularly of the prostate. These nutrients work by stopping cancer cells from growing, spreading, and invading other tissues. They take away cancer's passport, so it can't wreak havoc in other parts of your body.

Phytates kill bad cells and spare the good. Antioxidants called phytates also keep cancer cells from spreading, say colon and breast cancer studies. And it's not just through antioxidant effects. Phytates also support your immune system and fight inflammation, a longtime cancer culprit.

The best part is phytates appear to go after cancerous cells, leaving normal cells alone.

Fiber cuts back cancer risk factors. Fiber, particularly insoluble fiber, fights factors that raise your chances of developing tumors.

The roughage travels to your gut where it feeds good bacteria. These guys create beneficial short-chain fatty acids, which help lower colon cancer risk.

Fiber also fends off prostate cancer by fighting inflammation and balancing certain hormones.

Pair the perfect diet with easy movement for strength and balance

Exercise and a plant-based diet are a perfect pair. Just ask the only U.S. male weightlifter to make it to the 2016 Olympics — vegan Kendrick Farris. But you don't have to become a bodybuilder to get the benefits of a good work-out. Try low-impact exercises — ideal for everyone over 50.

Think of these as activities that don't place stress on your joints. Walking, bicycling, swimming, and using an elliptical get your heart pumping and muscles working without putting so much pressure on your knees, hips, and back.

These types of exercises also improve balance and strength. In fact, activities such as yoga and tai chi may cut your risk of falling and injuring yourself. Tai chi reduced this risk by almost 50 percent in one study. Who knew striking a pose could help you sidestep a pitfall of aging.

4 smooth reasons to eat this humdinger of a dip

The Guinness world record for the biggest plate of hummus weighed in at more than 23,000 pounds. This headliner event took place in Lebanon, but the spread is famous all over the

world. Here are four reasons you might want a piece of
the action.

Whip up a delicious snack in a snap. Classic hummus is a
quick mix of puréed chickpeas, tahini, lemon juice, and garlic.
If you don't want to buy it ready-made, you can easily make
your own.

No tahini handy? Just replace the sesame seed paste with an
equal amount of peanut butter or Greek yogurt. Or simply
go without.

Go easy on your gut. As with other beans, you can wash away
some of the gas-causing sugars by soaking and rinsing.
Hummus goes the extra mile because the chickpeas, also known
as garbanzo beans, are mashed. This breaks down the fiber,
making it easier to digest.

Make dishes more nutritious. Hummus is not just a dip.
Switch it out for unhealthy condiments like mayonnaise, and
put it on sandwiches, wraps, or in foods like chicken salad.

Tease your taste buds. The best part of homemade hummus
is that you can tweak your flavors the way you want. In the
mood for more garlic and less lemon? It's up to you.

You don't have to stick to the traditional tang either. Give
classical hummus a tasty twist by adding pumpkin, sweet
potatoes, or beets.

Lemons

Lemonade — a sweet solution for kidney stones

This summertime refreshment has been the talk of the town for thousands of years. In ancient Egypt, people called it "qatarmizat," but you know it as lemonade. The benefits are nothing to pucker at. Drink a little each day, and you may lower your risk for kidney stones.

To understand how lemonade can kick stones to the curb, you have to dive deep into the relationship between sour lemons and your hardworking kidneys. Stones begin to grow in your kidneys when minerals and salts form crystals in your urine. But citrate in this icy refreshment breaks up stones before they ever make the agonizing journey through the narrow tube to your bladder. Here's how.

- A driving force behind kidney stones is supersaturation. This means your urine is swimming with too many salts and not enough fluids. It can happen if you get dehydrated, so keep lemon water on hand.

- Kidney stones can form if oxalate sticks to calcium while your kidneys make urine. Citrate binds with the calcium before it can pair up with oxalates to form crystals.

- Citrate can also bind to the crystals, which prevents them from growing into painful stones.

Up to 60 percent of people with calcium stones have low amounts of citrate in their urine. Even so, your odds of developing them aren't set in stone. And citrus fruits like lemons can help boost your citrate levels.

That's what researchers found when they asked people at risk for kidney stones to drink about 4 ounces of lemon juice daily. Urinary citrate levels went up significantly. Participants killed two birds with one stone — quenching thirst and supporting their kidneys.

While you enjoy your lemonade, don't be heavy-handed with the sugar bowl. Your kidneys don't like to be doused with the sweet stuff.

Add zing with zest — an 'ap-peel-ing' way to get more C

Just two tablespoons of lemon peel deliver about a fourth of the vitamin C you need each day. That means it's time to bust out your microplane grater! What? You don't have a zester? No problem. You can get cooking with tools you already have in your kitchen.

The key to a zippy zest is leaving that bitter white pith behind. Use a cheese grater, knife, or vegetable peeler to trim off strips of the colorful rind. Cut into thin strands or finely mince.

Have lemons now but need zest later? You can store it in a plastic bag up to three weeks in the freezer before it starts to lose flavor. When you're ready, take it out and sprinkle on pasta, add to baked goods, or mix into a sauce for a jazzed-up dish.

3 reasons lemons are going viral

Battling illness year-round can leave you sour. Put the squeeze on cold and flu symptoms with the fruit that packs a triple punch.

Strike the stomach bug with this secret ingredient. It came out of nowhere. The violent diarrhea, vomiting, and nausea — someone has norovirus. Also known as the stomach flu, this extremely contagious virus is the leading cause of tummy troubles in schools, cruise ships, and hospitals.

Just the thought of it has you ready to sterilize your home. As you reach for the disinfectants, notice many of these cleaners boast citric acid as an active ingredient. And for a good reason. The citrate in citric acid binds to the virus. This keeps it from making a cozy home inside your healthy cells, according to a recent study.

While scientists are still investigating if citric acid can slash symptoms, some people already swear by it. One virologist says three glasses of lime juice eased his symptoms. Another person claims several ounces of lemon juice a day kept the bug at bay.

"E-lemon-ate" colds faster with vitamin C. How often do you see roadside stands for boring orange juice? Fresh, tangy lemonade has the edge over OJ. And like all citrus juices, it's also packed with vitamin C to keep your immune system humming along.

But can it clobber a cold? Although past research on the topic has been up and down, a recent review reveals some encouraging news.

* In four British trials, vitamin C pared down the frequency of colds by 30 percent in men who were slightly deficient in the vitamin.

* Researchers found that people who took 200 milligrams (mg) of vitamin C each day throughout the study, then developed a cold, shortened the time they suffered

symptoms by 9 percent. The research showed you'll benefit most by getting vitamin C in your diet regularly, rather than waiting until you catch a cold.

- Higher doses of vitamin C had even better results, shortening cold length by as much as 19 percent, say multiple studies.

Easy way to ease symptoms. You'd need to eat about 4 1/2 large lemons to get the 200 mg of vitamin C daily that was shown to reduce cold symptoms. That will give your mouth quite a pucker! If you're constantly battling sniffles, sore throats, and coughs, talk to your doctor about trying a vitamin C supplement. An extra perk is that vitamin C may relieve respiratory troubles like asthma that are worsened by colds, experts say.

So keep sipping your lemon water, and add lemon slices to your meals to punch up the flavor. If you're blindsided by a cold, try this classic sore throat soother. Brew a hot cup of tea and add a dollop of honey and splash of lemon.

Citrus strikes a bitter blow against cancer

People use the word "lemon" to refer to cars with serious faults, but actual lemons are seriously fabulous. Here's why — this delicious citrus may be a natural way to fight cancer. Check out the juicy details.

Tart up your tumor defenses with antioxidants. Vitamin C is up to 10 times more successful at shutting down cancer growth than certain experimental drugs, according to scientists from the University of Salford in Manchester, England. This potent antioxidant paints a bullseye on cancer stem cells and kills them before they can multiply and fuel fatal tumors.

One large lemon packs about 44.5 milligrams of vitamin C. And when it comes to fighting cancer, studies show lemons are near the top of the food chain.

Scientists tested 11 common fruits to see which were best at stamping out liver cancer in a culture dish. They examined both antioxidant activity and the ability to stop cancer cells from growing. Two fruits rose to the top of the cancer-fighting list — cranberries and, you guessed it, lemons.

Taste the cancer cure found only in citrus. "If I ask why you should drink orange juice every day, almost everyone would say for vitamin C," says Dr. Ed Harris, who studied the effects of citrus on cancer at Texas A&M University. "That's true, but we also need to learn two new words — flavonoids and limonoids."

These nutrients give the fruits color and flavor, but they do much more behind the scenes. The duo nips cancer in the bud before it can form and puts a halt to cancer cells already in your body.

A healthy lemon tree can bear hundreds of pounds of fruit each year. Grow your own in a pot! Since they don't produce lemons for the first few years, start with a young plant. To keep your tree in tiptop shape, provide good drainage, plenty of sun, and steady fertilization.

Flavonoids are found in many fruits and veggies, including lemons. But limonoids stand out because they are unique to citrus. The juice, seeds, and peels contain about 40 types of limonoids.

So snack on more oranges, grapefruit, and lemons. The same nutrient that makes them taste bitter can also take a bite out of cancer.

Fresh ways to squeeze more juice from your fruit

The old tried-and-true methods of juicing lemons might still work for you. But try these twists on classic tips, and you may pull out more juice.

Get the juiciest fruit by picking lemons heavy for their size, tradition says. The new advice — look for lemons that give under pressure. It's a mark of thin skin and more juice.

The best way to store lemons is in a plastic bag in the fridge. But cold lemons are harder to squeeze. Roll them on the counter, goes the old wisdom. Here's a better idea. Microwave whole lemons for 20 seconds, and let them cool slightly before juicing. Easy peasy lemon squeezy.

Beat the blues with this 'scent-sational' yellow fruit

"I love the smell of lemons," says Cindy Maxwell, who works an office job from nine to five. "I keep a bottle of the essential oil at my desk to save me from that afternoon slump." Even if you don't spend eight hours a day in a cubicle, plunging moods and low concentration can strike at any time. The good news is, a solution may be just a sniff away.

Get a whiff of the good ol' days for a quick pick-me-up. Grab a lemon and take a deep breath. Does it bring back memories? Lemon meringue pie at your grandmother's house? Ice cold lemonade in the middle of summer? Smells and memories are intertwined.

The scent receptors in your nose send the tangy smell of lemons straight to your brain. Your noggin hangs onto the information.

And voilà — one smell can trigger a flood of memories. Experts think when you associate happy experiences with specific smells, the scent may whip up positive thoughts.

Boost alertness with a stimulating scent. The mood-boosting effects of lemons aren't just hearsay. Researchers asked 56 men and women to smell lemon oil, lavender oil, or plain old water. Time after time, the invigorating scent of lemons was best at keeping spirits high.

Lemon oil boosts the brain chemical norepinephrine, which is linked to alertness, attention, and stress. Unsurprisingly, low norepinephrine activity is linked to depression.

Wake up and smell the lemons — three easy ways. Don't limit lemons to when you're cooking in the kitchen. Add the fruity fragrance to your entire home any time you like.

- Put aromatherapy to practice by setting up a diffuser, adding a few drops of lemon essential oil to a cotton ball, or mixing scents in a spray bottle.

- Cut up citrus fruits and simmer them in a pot of water. The steam will release the aroma throughout the room.

- Make your own lemon potpourri. Dry lemon peels in the oven on the lowest setting. Put them in breathable pouches and spread the love.

Green cleaning — natural ways to say goodbye to hidden grime

Let's face it. Some things in your house are just hard to clean. Rather than neglect these mischief-makers, test out the cleaning power of lemons. They cut through stains and overcome odors to leave even the most overlooked places in your home fresh and clean.

Go at your garbage disposal from a new angle. Tossing lemons down the chute is a common way to freshen a smelly disposal. But have you ever pulled out the black rubber stopper or taken a peek at the splash guard? Gag. Clean the stinky, slimy rubber parts with a simple, two-ingredient paste — baking soda and lemon juice.

Slowly mix the lemon juice with baking soda to make a paste. Rub it on the surfaces of the splash guard, stopper, and gasket. Let the mixture sit for 10 to 15 minutes before you scrub-a-dub-dub and rinse. If the parts aren't removable, you can reach them with a toothbrush.

Launder away stains with a simple scrub. Underarm stains are the pits. But you don't have to toss out your white wardrobe. Scrub the stained area on white shirts, blouses, even dresses, with lemon juice and water.

If your clothes need a little more attention, soak the dingy fabric in a gallon of hot water and a half cup of lemon juice for an hour or more. Toss them into the washing machine and launder as usual. Not only will your clothes come out looking whiter and brighter, but you'll also get rid of any lingering odors.

Wave away a dirty kitchen eyesore. You open up the microwave to heat up your breakfast and — wham! You're hit with the unsightly view of your last nine meals. You've been putting off cleaning because it seems like such a daunting task. Really, all you have to do is follow these simple steps.

- Add a few lemon slices to a small bowl of water, and microwave for five minutes.

- Let the bowl sit for a few more minutes to allow the steam to loosen the gunk.

- Wipe away the muck, take a step back, and smile.

Destroy anthills with a natural blend

You may enjoy the scent of lemons, but the critters who share your backyard don't. That's because citrus peels are laced with natural pesticides that drive off creepy-crawlies like those unwelcome fire ants.

This pesticide is in the form of d-limonene, the colorless oil found in lemon peels that give them the classic citrus scent. It's good for you but toxic to fire ants.

You could make your own chemical-free ant killer with citrus essential oils. But for a cheaper alternative, use leftover citrus peels. Soak the rinds of three lemons in a gallon of water for 10 days. Make sure you cover it. Remove the peels, and drench the undisturbed anthills in the solution. It may take a few days to eliminate the colony.

Mangoes

Knock out cancer with a little mango magic

"To most enjoy a mango," said distinguished American chef James Beard, "one should probably eat it in a bathtub, or at the very least in private." He was, of course, referring to the fabulously juicy goodness you'll find inside any of the 1,000 varieties of this tropical delight.

The mango, originally from India, is the most widely consumed fruit in the world, thanks to its fresh flavor and versatility. You'll find it lending a hint of sweetness to salsas, smoothies, salads, and sorbets — although it is just as tasty in pork or rice dishes as it is in cobblers or cheesecakes.

Surprisingly, the mango is related to the cashew and pistachio but offers its own mix of stellar nutrients, like beta carotene, vitamin C, and fiber. Yet it's the natural compounds called polyphenols, known for their top-notch health benefits, that captured the attention of a team of food scientists in Texas.

They pitted mango polyphenol extracts against colon, breast, lung, leukemia, and prostate cancers. "The breast and colon cancer lines underwent apoptosis, or programmed cell

"Leaves of three, let it be" is the warning that helps you identify poison ivy and steer clear lest you break out in a blistery rash. Mangoes should come with a similar caution. Their skin contains the same toxin as poison ivy — urushiol. If you're sensitive, wear gloves to peel your mango before eating.

death," says Dr. Susanne Talcott, lead researcher. "Additionally, we found that when we tested normal colon cells side by side with the colon cancer cells, that the mango polyphenolics did not harm the normal cells."

Talcott and her team believe a specific group of polyphenols, called gallotannins, target cells on the verge of forming tumors and stop them from progressing to cancer.

Mangoes contain both large and small polyphenols, but since you don't absorb the large compounds as easily, they reach your intestines intact. This means colon cancer cells get a double whammy — small polyphenols attacking through your bloodstream and larger ones through the lining of your intestines.

When people think of superfoods, they usually go for those with the strongest antioxidant power. But Talcott argues mangoes, with their incredible anticancer punch, more than deserve the title.

Supermarket tango bags a just-right mango

You can't judge a mango by its color. Because the skin can vary from green to yellow, orange, and even red, depending on the variety, simply eyeballing the fruit is not a good measure of ripeness. You have to give it a squeeze. A ripe mango will be firm, but not hard.

Now sniff. Notice a sweet, fruity aroma, especially at the stem end? Then it's perfect.

Watch out for signs of overripeness, though — loose or wrinkled skin and a sour or alcoholic smell.

If you bring home a mango that's not quite ready, just let it sit on the counter for three to five days. To speed things up, place it in a paper bag.

Sweet treat beats midlife heat

If you can't stand the heat, get into the kitchen — and slice open a fresh, juicy mango. It's one of five fruits that will help cool off miserable hot flashes and night sweats.

Australian researchers studied the eating habits of more than 6,000 menopausal women over nine years. They found:

- those who ate high-fat and sugary meals suffered the most from these uncomfortable symptoms.

- fruit-eaters and women on a Mediterranean-style diet, which included salad greens, peppers, mushrooms, garlic, pasta, and red wine, experienced fewer episodes.

The cooling fruits? Pineapple, strawberries, melon, apricots, and — of course — mango.

Experts say what you eat affects your estrogen levels and can therefore keep "private summers" from consuming your life. The winning diet styles include lots of fiber and no trans fats from processed foods, which translates into lower and more stable estrogen levels. When you eat this way, you're also getting carbohydrate-rich foods that keep your blood sugar steady. And that's been linked to fewer hot flashes.

One refreshing way to cool off is to whip up a traditional mango smoothie known as an Indian lassi.

1 1/4 cups diced mango	1/2 cup light coconut milk
1/4 cup mango nectar	1/4 cup plain Greek yogurt
1/2 cup ice cubes	1 tablespoon honey
1 tablespoon lime juice	

Purée all ingredients in a blender. Top with ground pistachio nuts. Makes 2 cups.

Blood sugar control: go mad for mangoes

Struggling with a few too many pounds or high blood sugar? Don't snub the mango. Sure, it's sweet, coming in at a little over 100 calories per cup. But two studies presented by researchers at the Federation of American Societies for Experimental Biology found that mango is still a "go-go."

First, 20 adults, each with a body mass index (BMI) in the obese range, ate 10 grams of dried mango every day for 12 weeks. That's equal to about two-thirds of a cup of fresh mango. At the end of the study, their blood sugar levels were lower than when they started, while their weight was unaffected.

Hoping to confirm these findings, the research team later tested the same strategy on people suffering from prediabetes. This is a condition where your blood sugar level is higher than normal but not yet high enough to be classified as type 2 diabetes. Again, mangoes had a positive effect on glucose levels. Getting prediabetes under control is critical if you want to prevent damage to your heart, blood vessels, and kidneys.

> Add mango to your next beef or pork marinade, then sit back and wait for the compliments to roll in. Your meat will turn out fork-tender, thanks to a certain protein-digesting enzyme in the fruit that breaks down tough tissues.

Slip the tasty mango into your diet as often as you can. You'll pack in nutrients and do your blood sugar some good at the same time.

Manuka honey

Sweet solution for wounds that won't heal

Honey may be the perfect addition to a cup of tea, but did you know it can also treat sores, burns, and many types of open wounds? It's an ancient remedy that is not just an old wives' tale. Certain types of honey — especially one called manuka — kill bacteria festering inside wounds and help your body heal naturally.

Manuka honey is made by bees that feed on the flowers of manuka trees in New Zealand and Australia. While it may taste sweet, it's no ordinary honey. Manuka is packed with special properties that make it ideal for treating wounds.

- All honey, including manuka, draws fluid up from the bottom of the wound to its surface. This keeps the area moist, which helps it heal.

- Normally, bacteria love growing in these moist places, but manuka contains a secret weapon, called methylglyoxal. This is the active ingredient which fights bacteria.

- Manuka is also a natural anti-inflammatory. While other honeys can cool inflammation, manuka is more powerful, again thanks to methylglyoxal.

- Manuka can kick-start the healing process even in long-term, chronic wounds. Plus, it helps wounds heal faster than they would on their own.

Studies show manuka can tackle some of the toughest injuries, like these.

Chronic wounds. Long-lasting injuries often refuse to heal because bacteria have crept in and set up shop. The bacteria band together and build a film around themselves like a shield. Once that happens, antibiotics may not be able to break through.

Manuka can dissolve the film around even hard-to-kill bacteria like methicillin-resistant *Staphylococcus aureus* (MRSA), so the wound can finally mend.

Diabetic ulcers. Studies show even stubborn diabetic ulcers healed within three months when dressed with manuka honey. Still, have your doctor monitor you closely.

Bed sores. A study, published in the journal *Spinal Cord*, reported manuka honey cleared bacteria out of pressure ulcers in as little as one week, and completely healed them within a month.

Burns. Honey is proven to soothe the pain of minor burns, help them heal faster, and reduce scarring.

All this sounds great, but you can't just slather on some honey and expect a miracle. First, check with your doctor and make sure that manuka will actually help the kind of wound you have.

Next, get the right product. Yes, you can buy a jar of manuka honey, but you need a product labeled "medical-grade" which has been gamma-irradiated to make it sterile and safe for wounds.

Ask your doctor which type of product you should use. For instance, you can buy medical-grade manuka as an ointment or as a bandage with honey in it. And find out if you will need your doctor or nurse to help change the dressing on your wound while it heals.

Buzzworthy news: only magnificent manuka will do

Don't smear supermarket honey on a cut and expect it to heal. Researchers analyzed regular table honeys, including clover and orange blossom, for bacteria-fighting power. Ten of the 18 honeys tested had no effect on bacteria at all. Worse, some honeys actually contained bacteria that could infect a wound.

Experts warn that honeys made for eating are not evaluated or regulated the way medical-grade honey is. What's more, medical-grade honey is sterilized with gamma rays. This kills any bacteria in it without destroying its healing properties. Edible honeys may have been sterilized with heat, which wipes out their bacteria-killing compounds.

Liquid gold takes the sting out of cancer treatments

An explosion of lifesaving cancer therapies bring new hope, but, in many cases, also new side effects. Enter honey. Evidence shows it can help heal some damage caused by radiation and chemotherapy.

Dermatitis. Radiation harms skin cells, which can leave you with itchy, red, and painful dermatitis. In separate studies, women undergoing radiation for breast cancer:

- had less severe dermatitis if they applied manuka honey to their skin twice a day, beginning the first day of radiation.

- found honey-infused gauze eased pain, itching, and irritation, and helped skin heal faster after radiation.

Talk to your doctor about using medical-grade, manuka-infused ointments and bandages such as products marketed under the brand name MEDIHONEY.

Mucositis. Chemotherapy and radiation may kill cancer cells, but they also kill the benign cells lining your mouth, throat, and digestive tract. The result is mucositis — painful ulcers that can make it hard to eat, drink, or simply swallow.

Multiple studies show that eating honey can help prevent mucositis in people getting radiation for head and neck cancer. Most found relief by taking four teaspoons of honey three times a day throughout the course of their treatment. To try it yourself, swish each mouthful for up to two minutes, then slowly swallow it. You can use manuka honey, but you don't have to. Many types will work.

In a surprising twist, researchers recently stumbled upon an unexpected benefit from a honey and coffee combination. They found a homemade brew healed chemo-induced mucositis better than steroids and better than honey mixed with water. Discuss this remedy with your doctor before you try it.

- Brew strong coffee made from 10 ounces of water with about six tablespoons of instant coffee.

- Stir in about one cup of local or manuka honey.

- Sip then swallow three teaspoons of this mixture every three hours for one week.

Since heat destroys some of the healing properties of honey, let your coffee cool to room temperature before adding the honey.

Safeguard your honey hoard

You probably pop some foods in the fridge out of habit, not necessity. But honey hates being cold! Refrigeration just makes it crystallize faster, and microwaving it to melt the crystals can destroy the healing compounds in manuka honey.

Instead, store it in a cool, dark cabinet away from direct sunlight. Never close to a heat source, like above the stove or beside the oven, either. If it does crystallize, place the jar in warm water and stir the honey until it dissolves.

Check out these 14 other whole foods you should never refrigerate.

Basil	Bread
Coffee grounds	Fresh garlic
Fresh ginger	Ground herbs and spices
Melons	Onions
Potatoes	Tomatoes
Winter squash	Unripe avocados
Unripe plums	Unripe bananas

These seven foods don't mind being cold, but you don't have to refrigerate them.

All-purpose flour	Apples
Citrus	Cucumbers
Nuts	Oils
Peanut butter	

Honey trap: don't fall for fake manuka

This honey is one hot ticket. And it's pricey. For these reasons, you have to be wary of impostors. Dishonest sellers may try to pass off their regular honey as manuka, or claim that a weak brand of manuka is stronger than it really is. Don't fall prey to scams like these.

Some manuka is not as strong as it claims. Researchers bought three brands of manuka honey and tested their antibacterial strength. One brand was a medical-grade product called MEDIHONEY, while the other two were regular jars of manuka from a supermarket. Only the medical-grade honey was as strong as it claimed.

Not surprisingly, the stronger, medical-grade manuka did the best job of fighting methicillin-resistant *Staphylococcus aureus* (MRSA) and other bacteria.

And some isn't manuka at all. A British newspaper went shopping online and at supermarkets around London. They bought a variety of regular (not medical-grade) manuka honeys, then had them all tested at an independent laboratory. Turns out, many honeys labeled "manuka" were knockoffs.

Buy with confidence. Batches of manuka are rated on the amount of bacteria-fighting compounds they contain. In theory, you can tell how pure — and beneficial — your jar of manuka is by the Unique Manuka Factor (UMF) number on its label. According to the Unique Manuka Factor Honey Association (UMFHA) of New Zealand, the number inside the logo represents "the unique signature compounds characteristic

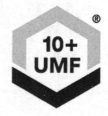

of this honey which ensure purity and quality." That includes methylglyoxal. Anything rated 10 and higher should be strong enough to fight bacteria.

If you plan to use it on wounds, buy medical-grade manuka products approved by the Food and Drug Administration. If you want to eat it as a health food, look for jars of manuka that carry the UMF rating logo. When you see this logo, you'll also know the honey was tested by the UMFHA, is real manuka honey, and is as strong as it claims to be. You can find trustworthy sellers through the UMFHA website at *umf.org.nz/umf-members*.

Smoothie sensation with a tropical twist

Honey is just too good to reserve for the medicine cabinet. So be sure your pantry always has a jar, ready to sweeten a batch of muffins or that cup of tea. Here's one refreshing idea that will have you going back for more.

   2 cups diced, peeled ripe papaya

   2 1/2 cups diced pineapple

   1/4 cup lime juice

   1/4 cup honey

Combine ingredients in a blender. Blend until slushy and almost smooth. Add more honey if needed for taste. Pour mixture over cracked ice in a tall glass. Garnish each with a mint sprig and a pineapple cube. Makes 5 servings at 115 calories per serving.

Mint

Go menthol — 5 fresh ways to make use of mint

This ancient herb is amazingly easy to grow, and good for so much more than cooking. From improving digestion to repelling pests, mint packs a mean punch against your biggest bothers. The secret ingredient — menthol.

A cool way to make muscle pain disappear. The smell and feel of menthol is unmistakable. It's what causes that cool feeling when you eat peppermint candies or brush with minty toothpaste.

Menthol blocks your cold-sensing nerves. That's how it eases pain and why it's an active ingredient in many traditional rub-on pain-relief products.

Try a menthol cream or gel to soothe muscles and joints. For a natural twist, add a few drops of spearmint or peppermint oil to your favorite carrier oil or lotion and rub-a-dub-dub.

Head throbbing? Soothe it with a minty blend. Menthol also helps relieve both tension headaches and migraines. So instead of popping a painkiller every time a headache crops up, try dabbing one of these mixtures on your forehead.

- Add peppermint essential oil to a carrier oil like sweet almond. It will tone down the blend so it doesn't irritate your skin.

- If you don't have an oil, make some peppermint tea. Wait for it to cool, then apply with a wash cloth.

Tea takes the heat out of sunburn. Summer fun can come to a standstill when sunburn comes to town. But menthol calms a sunburn by cooling and refreshing your skin. To take the sting out of the burn, make a strong peppermint tea. Apply the cooled mixture to the burned area with a cloth.

Mint cools off cold symptoms. Menthol relieves your cough and sore throat by interfering with cold-sensing nerves and the cough reflex. But it does more than that. It also acts as a decongestant, thinning mucus and breaking up phlegm.

Make a mint steam treatment for instant relief. Boil a pot of water, turn off the heat, and add a few drops of peppermint essential oil. Then lean over the pot, and breathe in.

Breathe better for a better workout. Menthol could be the secret to exercising longer and harder. It opens up your airways, increasing the amount of oxygen that gets to your body.

Researchers agree. Participants in one study performed a treadmill exercise test. Then for 10 days they drank a daily bottle of water with a drop of peppermint oil. When they retook the test, they ran significantly longer.

But as they say — don't try this at home. You should always talk to your doctor first before you swallow essential oils.

Pick peppermint for an instant stomach soother

Ah, the post-dinner peppermint. It's not just for fresh breath, you know. Mint also appeals to your senses to cure your biggest tummy troubles. Check out these three ways to wave goodbye to digestive woes.

Sip your way to IBS relief. Stomach pain, diarrhea, and constipation. It sounds like the lyrics to the Pepto-Bismol song. But it's actually the symptoms of irritable bowel syndrome (IBS), a disease that targets the large intestine.

But experts say mint calms the muscles in your digestive tract, particularly those that can cause spasms in the main part of your large intestine.

To test the theory, a small group of volunteers took two enteric-coated capsules containing 225 milligrams of peppermint oil twice a day for a month. Peppermint oil helped settle stomach pain, diarrhea, constipation, and more.

> The burning question — will peppermint cause heartburn? It's possible. Mint can relax the sphincter that keeps acid in your stomach and out of your esophagus, causing that burning sensation. If you have acid reflux, your doctor may suggest coated capsules.

Most studies used capsules, but experts say peppermint tea might work too. Pour a spot of tea, or blend some fresh leaves into a smoothie.

Rub out gas grief with an essential massage. Mint tea and capsules may also help gas, bloating, and indigestion by improving the flow of bile through your pipes. This helps speed and ease digestion.

Want to go a step further? A combo of essential oil and a little bit of pressure may be just what you need to get things moving along.

Mix five drops of peppermint essential oil with a tablespoon of a carrier oil. Rub clockwise on your tummy — up the right side, across just under the diaphragm, down the left, and across your lower abdomen.

Take a whiff to calm a churning gut. Tea and capsules are handy, but what if you're too nauseated to eat? Enter aromatherapy.

Researchers analyzed folks suffering from post-surgery nausea. Participants used a nasal inhaler that contained peppermint oil. In just two minutes, they reported less nausea.

Sniff the essential oil straight from the bottle. Or crush up some fresh peppermint leaves and take a deep breath.

Tag team your taste buds with cool mint pairings

Hundreds of varieties of mint, one dish. How do you choose? Many mints are interchangeable, while others offer a distinct flavor. If you don't know where to begin, test out these options to find your favorite combos.

Type	Try it with
Apple mint	salads, sauces
Chocolate mint	desserts
Ginger mint	vinaigrettes, soups
Orange mint	salsa, salads
Peppermint	tea, desserts
Spearmint	meats, vegetables

If the package at the store says mint, it's probably spearmint. This kind is popular for cooking and the easiest to find at your local superstore. The simplest way to get access to other tasty varieties is to grow your own herb garden.

Keep your mind razor sharp — morning, noon, and night

A morning or afternoon slump can derail the best-laid plans. Perk up with tasty peppermint tea, say researchers from Northumbria University's Department of Psychology.

They asked 180 volunteers to drink either chamomile, peppermint, or hot water. And they tested their brain power and mood before and after drinking.

The peppermint raised their spirits and sharpened their minds, improving their long- and short-term memory. The drink also made them more alert.

"Peppermint has a reputation for being psychologically or mentally alerting. It picks you up and makes you feel a little bit brighter," says Dr. Mark Moss, leader of the study. "We found that those people who drank the peppermint tea had better long-term memory. They were able to remember more words and pictures that they had seen."

That's a boon for older Americans who want to protect their memory. Try adding a delicious cup of peppermint tea to your morning, afternoon, or evening meal — or better yet, to all three.

3 really good reasons to plant it in a pot

Ready to join the herb "move-mint"? Place your plants in pots rather than in your garden and reap three cool benefits.

Close by when you need 'em. Potted mint plants are easy to move to your porch or deck. That's handy when you want to grab a few leaves to make tea or toss in a favorite recipe.

Contains the love. Mint loves to spread. Give it lots of water and sun, and its long runners can take over your garden. Put it in a pot, and you're good to go.

Repels irritating pests. The ants go marching home again when they encounter this sweet-smelling spice. Bees and mice also dislike mint. You can move the plant around where you need it the most.

Monounsaturated fats

MUFAs and metabolic syndrome: 3 ways a smart fat makeover nixes this risky mix

It's not only how much. It's what kind. That's the golden rule when it comes to fat in your diet. In fact, one of the biggest mistakes you can make is to cut out all fat from the foods you eat. Your body needs it to function — for muscles to do their work and for your intestines to absorb important nutrients.

The fat fallacy — not all are created equal. But it is true, certain fats have a dark side. You need to get smart about them so you can make healthy decisions.

Type of fat	Health facts	Common sources
Saturated Fatty Acids (SFAs)	• considered unhealthy because they contribute to high levels of bad cholesterol in your blood • linked to conditions like cancer, high blood pressure, type 2 diabetes, atherosclerosis, obesity, and stroke	• animal fats • tropical plant oils like coconut and palm • whole milk products • coconut
Polyunsaturated Fatty Acids (PUFAs)	• can improve blood cholesterol levels • may help lower your risk of type 2 diabetes	• corn, soybean, and safflower oils • fish and fish oil • walnuts • pumpkin and sunflower seeds • flaxseed

Type of fat	Health facts	Common sources
Monounsaturated Fatty Acids (MUFAs)	• can help lower your LDL (bad) cholesterol levels, which reduces your risk of heart disease and stroke • may benefit insulin levels and blood sugar control	• olives and olive oil • canola oil • sesame seeds and sesame oil • avocados • almonds, cashews, hazelnuts, macadamias, pecans, and pistachios • peanuts, peanut butter, and peanut oil

MUFAs challenge a metabolic meltdown. Eat them in place of unhealthy saturated fats for your heart's sake, but also because MUFAs battle a deadly combination of conditions called metabolic syndrome.

Fast becoming a global epidemic, metabolic syndrome affects more than a third of all adults in the United States alone. It puts you at a much greater risk of heart disease, diabetes, and stroke. You officially suffer from metabolic syndrome if you have three or more of the following:

• Abnormal cholesterol or triglyceride levels. Low "good" HDL cholesterol, with readings below 40 milligrams per deciliter of blood (mg/dL) for men and 50 mg/dL for women. Blood triglyceride levels of 150 mg/dL or higher.

• Excess belly fat. A waist circumference of 40 inches or more for men, and 35 inches or more for women.

• High blood pressure. Readings higher than 130/85 mmHg.

• High blood sugar. A fasting glucose of 100 mg/dL or greater.

You already know monounsaturated fats help manage cholesterol, but here are some fascinating facts about how they tackle
the other big three factors of metabolic syndrome.

Give your diet an oil change to whittle your middle. When it
comes to losing stubborn belly fat, nothing axes those inches
like monounsaturated fats.

One type, called oleic acid, releases a hunger-fighting super-
substance in your small intestine that triggers a feeling of
fullness — so you don't want to snack all the time. And recent
studies show MUFAs also fire up a fat-burning process in your
cells that keeps dangerous fat from building around your waist.

Beat high blood pressure without drugs. Study after study
shows olive oil, especially rich in oleic acid, consistently lowers
BP. In fact, research published in the *Archives of Internal Medicine*
showed blood pressure was controlled so well in a group taking
olive oil, their need for medicine was cut almost in half. That
means you could say so long to nasty drug side effects.

Make the switch to control blood sugar. Swap out the unhealthy
saturated fats in your diet for healthier unsaturated ones, and
research shows you can significantly
reduce your HbA1c, your average
blood sugar level for the past two to
three months.

> Monounsaturated,
> polyunsaturated, or
> saturated — regardless
> of type, every fat gram
> contains nine calories.

Experts explain it this way. Your
intestines secrete a particular
hormone, called glucagon-like
peptide-1 (GLP-1), that boosts insulin sensitivity. MUFAs ramp
up GLP-1 and so help your body naturally fight off diabetes.

Buyer beware — the wheels of crime are greased with olive oil

It could be a dramatic TV mini-series — shady, underworld group makes millions tampering with global product. Unfortunately, this is no fictional script, but the face of food fraud in the 21st century.

Fake olive oil? Who would have thought it. Yet this ongoing multinational scam has left foodies and home chefs scratching their heads. Whether their oil was diluted with a cheap substitute like soybean or corn oil, contaminated with potentially harmful chemicals, or simply labeled as higher quality oil than it actually was — who could tell?

Since there's no single standard or organization that guarantees quality of imported olive oil, some industry experts recommend you simply buy from reputable California producers. This state, which grows 99 percent of U.S. olives, recently passed the Grade and Labeling Standards for Olive Oil, Refined-Olive Oil and Olive-Pomace Oil.

Visit the California Olive Oil Council online at *cooc.com* for more information about their certification process.

Change your fat, change your mind

Bread dipped in rich, fruity olive oil instead of slathered with butter. Creamy avocado spread on your sandwich rather than cheese or mayonnaise. A sprinkle of almonds on your salad in place of bacon bits. Every time you make this kind of swap-out — replacing saturated fats (SFAs) with monounsaturated fats

(MUFAs) — you help your brain stay younger, stronger, and, well, happier.

Your brain on bacon. Your brain is 60 percent fat. Not the kind that plumps you up. Rather the fat molecules that are the major building blocks of cell membranes. These wrap around and insulate the delicate parts of nerve cells in your brain that communicate with other cells. Pretty important stuff.

The MUFAs you get from foods like olive oil, avocados, and almonds help keep these cell membranes strong yet flexible, protecting your brain from age-related damage.

On the other hand, a study published in the journal *Neuropsychopharmacology* found that eating too many foods rich in saturated fats damages the way your brain responds in various situations, perhaps by causing inflammation.

And that's why every swap-out is so important.

Think faster, remember better. During a four-year study of 6,000 women, researchers at Harvard University discovered those who ate the most MUFAs scored higher on tests of brain function and memory than women who ate saturated fats.

> No one thinks of it as juice. But, technically, olive oil is juice from the fruit of the olive tree. Bet you didn't know olives were a fruit, either.

Attack Alzheimer's at the source. Cholesterol buildup in your arteries plays a major role in developing Alzheimer's disease (AD). And saturated fats are major baddies when it comes to cholesterol. In addition, these same fats can damage the blood brain barrier, a layer of cells that protects your brain from harmful substances.

When researchers out of Rush University Medical Center in Chicago reviewed numerous studies on dietary fat and the brain, they found the risk of AD was higher when diets included saturated fats and lower when diets were rich in monounsaturated fats.

Feel a little groovy. Fine-tune the type of fat you eat and you could wind up happier. A study pitting two diets against each other — essentially SFAs versus MUFAs — revealed those eating the more healthy MUFAs felt less anger and hostility than the other group.

Liquid gold for beautiful skin

Brown spots, wrinkles, and sagging skin are the red flags of sun damage. But that doesn't have to describe you.

A study of almost 3,000 people showed that eating more monounsaturated fatty acids from olive oil lowered the risk of severe sun damage in both men and women. Two teaspoons or more a day will give you the best results.

While this is a delicious idea, there are plenty of other ways olive oil can help your skin.

- Soften hands by first rubbing in olive oil, then scrubbing with sugar. Rinse well.

- Dab just a drop onto dry, chapped lips.

- Soak your fingers in a bowl of warm olive oil for about 10 minutes, and say bye-bye to ragged cuticles.

- Add two to three tablespoons to a warm, soaking bath for all-over softness. Just take care when climbing out of the tub. It could be slippery.

Low-fat eating: a surprising vitamin thief

You're committed to lunchtime salads. You pass on potatoes and opt for cauliflower. You just say no to pie and yes to fruit. In short, you're doing everything you can to eat healthy. Or are you?

Remember, making smart food choices is about more than calories. It's about lutein, lycopene, beta carotene and zeaxanthin. Vitamins A, D, E, and K. In short, it's about the nutrients in those delicious fruits and vegetables you've come to know and love. And it's about the fact you could be sabotaging all your hard work by cutting out the fat.

"If you want to utilize more from your fruits and vegetables, you have to pair them correctly with fat-based dressings," says Mario Ferruzzi, Purdue associate professor of food science. "If you have a salad with a fat-free dressing, there is a reduction in calories, but you lose some of the benefits of the vegetables."

For example, build a spinach salad with sweet red peppers, carrots, and tomatoes. Congratulations, you're about to enjoy a meal loaded with nutrients that can cut your risk of several serious conditions such as cancer, heart disease, and macular degeneration. But top this salad with just a drizzle of vinegar or a simple squirt of lemon juice and your body can't absorb these fat-soluble nutrients.

According to Ferruzzi, monounsaturated fats (MUFAs), like olive oil, are the best choice for salad dressing, if you want to get the most nutritional bang for your buck.

Check out the following easy, homemade vinaigrette that is full of flavor and one oh-so-important MUFA.

1/4 cup extra virgin olive oil

1/4 cup balsamic vinegar

1/4 cup orange juice

2 tsp minced fresh ginger

1 tsp minced fresh thyme

1/4 tsp salt

1/8 tsp black pepper

Combine all ingredients and whisk together vigorously. Store in the fridge for up to a week. Add 1/4 cup plain Greek yogurt if you prefer your dressing a little creamier.

The mighty olive: 3 little-known reasons to fry your heart out

Fried foods healthy? It's possible — as long as you fry in olive oil.

Bring on the old switcheroo. Any time you fry, components of the frying oil soak into your food. It's just common sense then to make a good-for-you choice, like virgin olive oil (VOO), rich in monounsaturated fatty acids (MUFAs). In studies, researchers report after lean fish were pan-fried in VOO, their MUFA content was two to six times higher than before frying.

Because fat also transfers the other way, from food to oil, olive-oil-fried meat, chicken, and fish ended up with lower levels of unhealthy saturated fatty acids. What a bonus!

Olive oil withstands the heat. All oils will oxidize and hydrogenate some, if repeatedly heated to very high temperatures. That means they undergo a slight chemical change making them dangerous in your body. But the MUFAs in olive oil resist these changes, and because olive oil has a high smoke point, it won't break down at frying temperatures.

Frying hangs on to those nutrients. Frying is usually a pretty quick process, with the core of your food not reaching as high a temperature as the outside layers. Because of this, the majority of vitamins don't break down or oxidize as they would during other cooking methods.

Remember, too, certain vitamins, like thiamine, riboflavin, B6, and C, are called water-soluble — they dissolve in water. So naturally you'll lose more of them when you boil foods, and fewer when you fry. Take a look at how choices you make in the kitchen affect how healthy your dishes end up.

Cooking method	% loss of water-soluble vitamins
boiling	35 - 60
roasting	10 - 47
steaming	10 - 25
microwave cooking	5 - 25
stewing	10 - 12
grilling	10 - 12
baking	10 - 12
pressure cooking	5 - 10
frying	7 - 10

Pineapple

Build your bones with a tropical treat

Would you pay $8,000 for a single pineapple? Hundreds of years ago, kings and queens paid through the nose just to get a taste of this exotic fruit. Because pineapples were so difficult to grow outside of the tropics, they became symbols of wealth and luxury throughout Europe.

Now scientists realize pineapples have a lot more to offer than great flavors. And if you knew all the health benefits of this tropical fruit, you might think they actually are worth their weight in gold.

Pineapples are loaded with a mineral called manganese. And if it isn't already high on your list of essential nutrients, it probably should be. Manganese plays a vital role in building your skeleton, but some experts think four out of every 10 people don't get enough of it. And because your bones are always being broken down and rebuilt, running short on any bone-building nutrients can cause osteoporosis.

The core of a pineapple is tough to eat and messy to remove. But if you have a cookie or biscuit cutter on hand, you'll have perfect pineapple rings in no time. Just peel and slice the pineapple, then carefully press your cookie cutter down on each slice to remove the core.

People usually think of calcium as being the only thing you need to ward off this serious disease, but manganese might be just as important. A study found women who took a

5-milligram supplement of manganese along with copper, zinc, and calcium helped stop bone loss. Researchers think manganese helps your bones by kick-starting the chemical messengers in charge of building strong bones and cartilage.

Pineapple is an easy and delicious way to get your fill of manganese. A single cup of this fruit contains 76 percent of your daily recommended dose.

Bromelain bites back against inflammation and clotting

When you take a bite out of a pineapple, it's biting you back — sort of. This fruit is chock-full of an enzyme called bromelain that attacks proteins. It's so powerful, bromelain is used to tenderize the toughest cuts of meat.

But this naturally occurring chemical can do so much more than marinate your next pot roast. Researchers think this unique chemical helps you get the upper hand in your battles against arthritis and blood clots.

Put arthritis pain in the past with this exotic enzyme.
Bromelain is a powerful anti-inflammatory, so researchers think it could help curb the pain and swelling caused by osteoarthritis. Researchers found bromelain works by blocking the chemicals in your body that trigger painful swelling and inflammation.

In a recent study, 30 people with chronic osteoarthritis of the jaw were divided into three groups. They either received a bromelain-based enzyme cocktail, a prescription nonsteroidal anti-inflammatory drug (NSAID), or a combination of both. At the end of the study, researchers found bromelain alone treated arthritis pain just as well as the NSAID. And when people took both, the treatment was even more effective.

People in this study took 180 milligrams of bromelain a day — way more than you can get from a pineapple. Every little bit helps, but if you really want to go all in, look for bromelain supplements online or at your local store.

Just be sure to talk to your doctor if you eat pineapple regularly or plan to take a bromelain supplement. This enzyme can cause dangerous side effects when mixed with some prescription drugs, including blood thinners, amoxicillin and tetrocycline antibiotics, and sedatives.

Bromelain leads the charge against blood clots. If you get a paper cut, nick yourself shaving, or scrape your knee, your body needs a way to repair the damage. That's where your platelets come in. Whenever these special blood cells detect damage, they clump together to start the healing process.

But sometimes this process can go haywire, and platelets will clot inside your blood vessels for no apparent reason. That can result in dangerous blood clots, which may set you up for a heart attack, stroke, or other serious health issues.

> The bromelain in pineapple not only breaks down proteins like chicken and beef, it can attack the proteins in your mouth and cause sores and swelling. Small amounts of pineapple are fine, but be careful not to overdo it. And don't worry about cooked or canned pineapple — heat destroys bromelain.

The good news is, scientists think bromelain can help you bust up blood clots. While they haven't tested this enzyme on humans yet, the early signs are promising. Test tube studies suggest bromelain stimulates an enzyme called plasmin, which your body uses to break apart the protein holding blood clots together.

If you're already taking prescription blood thinners, be careful how much pineapple you eat. Because bromelain also keeps your blood from clotting, you'll be at significantly more risk for bruising or bleeding.

How to pick the perfect pineapple

Pineapples stop ripening the second they are plucked from the plant, so you have to know exactly what to look for at the grocery store. Here are a few tips to help you take home the sweetest pineapples.

Don't get confused by color. Contrary to popular belief, a pineapple's color doesn't tell you anything about ripeness. Even green ones might be nice and sweet.

Make sure it passes the pluck test. Look for pineapples with bright green leaves and give them a tug. If the leaves are easy to pull out, it's a good sign.

Give it a squeeze. Pineapples should be firm, but the fruit should still have a slight give. If it's too hard or too mushy, try a new one.

Trust your nose. Ripe pineapples smell nice and sweet. Fruit with a sour smell is probably rotten.

Pistachios

Crunch time — defy diabetes with a tasty snack

Were you born before the 1980s? Then you probably remember red pistachios. Producers dyed them scarlet to hide the splotchy shell color that came from the harvesting methods of the times. But nowadays it's much easier to understand how they got the nickname "the green almond." In fact, the colorful hues are the reason experts give pistachios the green light for battling health hurdles like diabetes.

Pistachios are a culinary delight, brightening up even the dullest desserts and dinners. And they owe their surprising pop of color in part to antioxidants.

Groups of antioxidants called flavonoids and carotenoids are the masterminds behind pistachios' nutty health benefits. Add in a combo of healthy fats and fiber, and you've got the perfect recipe for balanced blood sugar. That's what scientists found in a recent study published in *Diabetes Care*.

- More than 50 people with prediabetes followed two diets, each for four months. The food selections had similar amounts of calories, protein, fiber, and healthy fats. The difference — one diet called for about 100 kernels of pistachios each day.

- The pistachio diet lowered blood sugar and insulin levels, which helped improve insulin resistance and other risk factors for diabetes. Your body needs steady levels of insulin to balance your blood sugar so your energy levels don't crash during the day.

The study was partly funded by the American Pistachio Growers. But studies show other nuts are good for high blood sugar, too. Grab a handful today to slash your risk for full-blown diabetes.

In a nutshell — pistachios lead to a lighter scale

Don't shy away from these nuts when you want to drop the pounds. Pistachios come preloaded with protein and fiber, keeping you fuller longer. No wonder they're called the skinny nut.

But with a crunch this tasty, it's easy to overindulge. Here's how to avoid scarfing down too many calories — always buy pistachios in the shell.

Folks who eat pistachios from shells toss back 41 percent fewer calories than those who eat them pre-shelled. That pile of empty pistachio shells reminds you how many you've eaten. Plus the effort it takes to shell the nuts slows you down, so you eat less.

Trade out other snacks, especially refined carbs, and let nuts take center stage. You may even lose more weight like the people in one three-month study who swapped pretzels for pistachios.

2 ways pistachios prompt good nights

Pistachios have always been pretty popular. They're mentioned in the first book of the Bible, after all. But this world-famous nut has a few secrets that often slip under the radar. For one, it's actually a seed. More importantly, pistachios give men support below the belt to make nights more enjoyable.

Boost blood flow with nature's Viagra. Erectile dysfunction — even the name is alarming. But for many men, trouble getting and keeping an erection is par for the course. It doesn't have to be. Just three weeks of eating less than a cup of pistachios a day improved bedroom business across the board in one small study.

A major cause of impotence is restricted blood flow, and pistachios may help in two ways.

- They're loaded with arginine. This amino acid relaxes blood vessels, keeping them flexible and encouraging blood to flow smoothly through your arteries.

- Cholesterol narrows your blood vessels, limiting blood flow. After eating pistachios, levels of bad cholesterol went down and the good kind went up.

Get better beauty sleep with fewer interruptions. Another way to ruin a perfectly good night is to interrupt sleep with visits to the bathroom. If you have an enlarged prostate, that's just the beginning. You may also experience stop-and-go urinating, a weak stream, and difficulty emptying your bladder completely.

But you'll take fewer nighttime bathroom trips when you get enough beta-sitosterol. According to a review of studies on men with lower urinary tract symptoms, this natural plant compound is a winner. It boosts urinary flow and helps you leave less urine in your bladder. Pistachios are one of the top sources of beta-sitosterol, with 61 milligrams in just 1 ounce of nuts.

> Tough nut to crack? You'll find at least one in every bag of pistachios. Here's what you do. Stick the nut in a garlic press, and squeeze until it cracks open. Voilà. If the shell isn't sealed tight, try a simpler technique. Slip an empty shell half into the crack, and twist.

Go nuts — boost blood flow to heal your heart

Lay all your blood vessels in a line, and you could circle the Earth four times. Veins, arteries, and capillaries cover a lot of ground. And to keep them working in tiptop shape, you need to make sure they stay healthy and flexible. Pistachios help you do that in two major ways.

Clear out buildup with a handful a day. Stockpiles of cholesterol block blood flow in your arteries, increasing your risk for heart problems. But pistachios could put a stop to all that, says a recent study published in *Nutrition*.

Researchers divided participants with raised cholesterol into two groups. For three months, both groups made healthy lifestyle changes, but only one got to eat pistachios.

Just one-third cup of these nutty treats a day bumped up good HDL cholesterol and lowered bad cholesterol. That means a healthy diet with good exercise habits — plus a handful of pistachios — can lead to healthier blood vessels.

Where does this protection come from? Antioxidants like lutein, beta carotene, and vitamin E.

Relieve pressure with the No. 1 nut. Nuts also take on high blood pressure. And pistachios are particularly qualified for the job.

A clever combo of healthy fats, phytosterols, and other nutrients work together to take the stress off your blood vessels, giving your heart a break.

A recent review of more than 20 studies, published in the *American Journal of Clinical Nutrition*, shows that eating pistachios lowers BP better than other nuts. Just don't undo the benefits by feasting on a bag of salted pistachios. Salt can hike up blood pressure without warning.

Prunes

Snack your way to a stronger skeleton

Prunes rocketed into the spotlight recently when scientists discovered they may prevent bone loss in astronauts exposed to radiation. What, you've never been to outer space? That's OK. The next superfood of the fruit world can also help build bones in those of you who are gravity-bound.

No matter where you are — from Crater Lake to a crater on the moon — your skeleton is a 24/7 construction zone. A demolition crew breaks down old bone while a rebuilding team forms a new frame. As you age, the building group slows down. This is why older folks often have fragile, more breakable bones.

But prunes, or dried plums if you prefer, might be able to change all that. Researchers are surprised at just how much disease-fighting power they have. The bone-healing potential comes from three mighty nutrients.

- **Antioxidants.** Prunes contain polyphenols that act as antioxidants to block bone loss and improve bone strength. Basically, they slow down the demolition crew and give help to the builders.

- **Vitamin K.** At 28.5 micrograms per serving of five prunes, these sweet treats are loaded with K. The powerful vitamin teams up with nutrients like calcium to help build stronger bones.

- **Boron.** No bones about it, boron is not as famous as its mineral cousin calcium. But it has an important place in bone health — extending how long vitamin D stays in your body. That's a big deal because vitamin D helps you absorb calcium.

Eat prunes, and you could build stronger bones in a matter of months, says a study partly funded by the California Dried Plum Board.

"Participants from our study maintained their bone mineral density by eating five to six dried plums per day," says Shirin Hooshmand, Ph.D., the lead researcher of the six-month study. "This can easily be achieved by snacking on dried plums or incorporating them into recipes."

Just eat a handful of these cheap, sweet fruits once a day. The best part — you may already have them in your fridge. Pair them up with other bone-building foods for a frame-fortifying diet. Try high-calcium foods like broccoli, canned salmon, and milk.

Dried plums: 1-step relief for constipation

A prune by any other name would taste as sweet. So when the California Prune Board changed the name to dried plums, most people weren't fazed. Industry leaders hoped to rid the fruit of its unfavorable link to bowel movements. But to the 60 million Americans who still suffer from chronic constipation, this link can be a life-changer.

Pitted prunes beat out popular laxative. What gives products like Metamucil the power to unclog your plumbing? Bulk-forming laxatives like psyllium. So for three weeks, scientists tested psyllium against a serving of dried plums twice a day.

The result? Ten daily prunes were better at making people "go" than psyllium supplements, say researchers. What a relief.

Clear pipes through the fiber effect. Fiber is the secret to stool movement. At 3.5 grams per serving, prunes are a good source of fiber — both soluble and insoluble.

- Soluble fiber attracts water, making stools larger, softer, and easier to pass.

- Insoluble fiber adds bulk to stools and helps waste pass more quickly through your system.

> Too much fiber all at once can unsettle your internal plumbing. To avoid cramping, diarrhea, and gas, gradually increase how much fiber you eat over a few weeks. And always drink plenty of water. Fiber needs fluids to keep things moving smoothly.

Before you head to the pharmacy to get rid of your digestive discomfort, do this. Turn down the dried fruit aisle and pick up the natural option that's both tasty and tough on constipation.

Find smooth sailing with sorbitol. "There's three things in this world that you need," said the late actor and comedian Robin Williams. "Respect for all kinds of life, a nice bowel movement on a regular basis, and a navy blazer." Thanks to prunes, you're already one step ahead.

Dried plums contain a sugar alcohol called sorbitol, which has fewer calories than regular sugar. That's because it's not fully absorbed by your intestines — the same reason it can have a laxative effect. Sorbitol draws water into your intestines, encouraging victorious visits to the bathroom.

Just remember that sorbitol can cause bloating, gas, and diarrhea in some people, especially those who suffer from irritable bowel syndrome. Take it slow until you know if it will help or hurt you.

Flavorful facelift — pep up prunes in just 10 minutes

Don't get yourself into a stew over trying to find fun ways to sneak prunes into dishes. Try this technique to transform these unglamorous dried fruits into deeply rich, silky soft delights. Here's what you need.

1 cup prunes

1 1/2 cups water

1/4 teaspoon cinnamon

1 small orange or 1/2 lemon (peeled and sliced)

Toss all ingredients into a pot, and bring to a boil. Cover and simmer 10 to 20 minutes or until plump and soft.

Eat the sweet-tart fruits over oatmeal, yogurt, waffles, or anything you can think of. Want more flavorful prunes with less work?

- Cover dried plums in orange juice and refrigerate overnight.

- Buy prunes prepackaged with a pop of flavor like cherry, lemon, and orange.

Prune away the pounds and shave an inch off your waistline

Say "prunes!" Nineteenth-century photographers actually used this instruction to capture those somber expressions you see in old portraits. It seems that prunes have given people a tight mouth for a long time. But researchers finally discovered how prunes can put a smile on your face, and it has everything to do with lowering that number on the scale.

How do prunes help you shed pounds? Scientists say fiber is the key. Fiber makes you feel full after a meal or snack. That means you'll be satisfied longer, which helps you eat less.

Researchers from the University of Liverpool put it to the test. After three months of adding prunes to their diets, obese participants who normally ate low-fiber diets lost 4.4 pounds and about an inch off their waists.

"In the long term prunes may be beneficial to dieters by tackling hunger and satisfying appetite — a major challenge when you are trying to maintain weight loss," says lead researcher Jo Harrold.

The downside is that participants had to eat 14 to 17 prunes a day, although researchers say they experienced no negative side effects. If you can't manage that many, berries, oatmeal, pears, and apples are all wholesome high-fiber choices.

Beat ticker troubles with a heart of stone

Peaches, apricots, and even cherries — these are all part of the stone fruit family. But none of them make a dried treat as finger-lickin' good as the plum. Dried plums aren't just tangy to your taste buds. They're also sweet to your ticker.

Drive down high cholesterol with fabulous fiber. Dietary fiber does a lot of fantastic things for your health, and lowering LDL cholesterol is one of them. Fiber keeps your body from absorbing too much cholesterol, so your levels don't skyrocket and cause problems like heart disease.

Upping fiber just 7 grams a day was associated with a 7 percent drop in stroke risk. You can get that amount in 10 prunes — just two servings a day.

Run-of-the-mill mineral axes high blood pressure. Eat more potassium. Scientists say it's a boon for blood pressure. A review of 33 studies on potassium intake showed that eating more of it lowered blood pressure and cut stroke risk by 24 percent. Maybe it's not so ordinary after all.

You can get more than a third of the potassium you need each day from a serving of prunes. Sneak more into your diet by trading out ingredients like raisins in your favorite snacks. Cut prunes into smaller bites, and toss them into cereal, granola, and oatmeal cookies. Yum.

Fruit face-off: do prunes have an edge over plums?

It takes 3 pounds of fresh plums to make 1 pound of prunes. With all that fruity goodness packed in, it's no wonder that — pound for pound and cup for cup — prunes offer some great nutritional benefits.

But it doesn't mean they always come out on top. Drying and juicing causes some vitamin and mineral loss. Take a look at the table to see how the nutrients stack up in a serving of each plum-yummy product.

Percent daily value in 1 serving

	5 prunes	1 cup of prune juice	2 plums
Fiber	14	10	8
Vitamin K	35	11	12
Potassium	10	20	7
Vitamin A	7	0	10
Calories	6	9	3

Percent Daily Values are based on a 2,000-calorie diet. Your daily values may be higher or lower depending on your calorie needs.

Pumpkin seeds

Squash bad moods with scrumptious seeds

Pumpkins boast a claim to fame in the most beloved fairy tale of all time. But they're good for more than elegant carriages. This member of the squash family also fights the blue funk. Pumpkin seeds contain two nutrients that boost serotonin, the feel-good chemical in your brain. Cue the happily ever after.

Revive your spirits with a mellow mineral. Magnesium — every organ in your body needs it, especially your brain. But many people just don't get enough from their diets.

Unfortunately, a simple deficiency in this mineral can bring you down with a wide array of symptoms — fatigue, anxiety, leg cramps, brain fog, mood swings, and headaches. But get your fill of magnesium and you can steady your serotonin levels, say experts.

The word serotonin gets thrown around a lot. Basically, it's a messenger in your brain that manages your mood by helping nerve cells communicate. No wonder low levels are linked to depression. But here's a surprising fact — magnesium makes antidepressants work better.

Experts recommend 400 milligrams (mg) of magnesium daily. Easily slip 38 percent of the magnesium you need into your diet with just an ounce of shelled pumpkin seeds. That's about 142 seeds — plenty for a mid-morning pick-me-up.

Carve out perfect pumpkin seeds for a yummy snack

Nothing says pumpkin season like a big, glowing jack-o'-lantern. But if you think carving out those triangle eyes is the best part, you don't know jack. Dig out the seeds, and add a little flavor by preparing them like a top chef.

First, grab a flat canning jar lid and scrape the seeds out. Then rinse the seeds and remove any pumpkin bits. Toss with seasoning to make it sweet, spicy, or savory. Favorite toppings include salt, honey and cinnamon, and butter and garlic. Follow either of these methods to make a tasty, crispy snack.

- Dry 'em. Layer seeds in a dehydrator at 115 degrees for one to two hours or in an oven on warm for three to four hours, stirring frequently.

- Roast 'em. Toss seeds with a tablespoon of olive oil. Spread them in a layer on a baking sheet. Roast at 300 degrees for 15 minutes or until seeds are lightly browned.

Amino acid axes anxiety. Magnesium is just one half of the pumpkin duo that fights down-in-the-dump feelings. The other warrior is tryptophan, an essential amino acid that helps make serotonin, which your body uses to make melatonin. Both of these brain chemicals play a supporting role in sleep and mood management.

In fact, as tryptophan levels go up, depression rates come down, say scientists who recently analyzed more than 29,000 cases of self-reported depression.

How does it work? Tryptophan is like that unlucky airplane passenger who doesn't get to go through the TSA PreCheck line.

While it's stuck waiting in the queue, all of the other PreCheck-eligible amino acids easily pass through security on their way to the departure gate, er, brain.

But wait, it gets better. When you eat a plant-based diet full of healthy carbohydrates, you get an added benefit. The carbs trigger a release of insulin, which diverts many amino acids to your muscles. Imagine all the other amino acids in front of tryptophan getting sent to a different line, leaving the path clear.

To get this process going, focus on eating plant foods like pumpkin seeds, sesame seeds, and walnuts that have a high tryptophan-to-protein ratio. The more tryptophan in the food, the more easily it will bypass the other amino acids and enter your brain.

The result — less anxiety and a calmer, more relaxed mood.

Hunger hack — transform ho-hum meals into crunchy creations

Leave the bread crumbs to Hansel and Gretel. Those refined carbs won't lead to a healthy home. Instead of breaded recipes, give your crusted meals an upgrade with crushed pumpkin seeds.

This crisp, nutty option isn't just healthier, it's also supremely tasty. Here's what you do. Coarsely chop hulled pumpkin seeds or grind them in a food processor, depending on the desired texture.

Mix the seeds with your favorite spices. Then coat your food of choice with a layer of the crunchy medley. It's an easy way to put a delicious new spin on crusted salmon or parmesan chicken. Who knew pumpkin seeds were so versatile?

Surprising way to pump up cancer protection

"There are three things I have learned never to discuss with people: religion, politics, and the Great Pumpkin," wrote Charles M. Schulz in his famous comic strip *Peanuts*. His beloved character Linus van Pelt may have had a rocky history in the pumpkin patch, but scientists have pushed this Halloween favorite back into the conversation.

That's because pumpkin seeds may lower your risk for breast cancer.

Researchers uncovered this exciting news when they reviewed studies of more than 8,000 postmenopausal women. They found that eating more pumpkin seeds, sunflower seeds, and soybeans was linked to lower breast cancer risk. But what's behind this delicious cancer buster?

All three foods contain phytosterols, natural compounds that help make up the structure of plant cell membranes. These chemicals interfere with your body's ability to produce and absorb LDL cholesterol. What does cancer have to do with cholesterol?

Experts say cholesterol may help cancerous cells grow and become more aggressive. Case in point — every 10-point drop in LDL cholesterol is linked to a 15-percent plunge in cancer risk, studies show. Basically, phytosterols get rid of the fodder that feeds cancer cells. That means you can fight heart problems and cancer worries with one yummy seed.

2 ways pepitas ward off prostate problems

Peter, Peter, pumpkin eater. Why was ol' Pete so fond of pumpkins? Perhaps he knew the seeds, often called pepitas, are packed with two ingredients that may protect his prostate.

Fix your flow with a natural plant compound. Frequent visits to the restroom. Inability to empty your bladder completely. Difficulty starting urination. Sound familiar? These are all symptoms of benign prostatic hyperplasia, or prostate enlargement. But how can you put the stream situation to rest? Beta-sitosterol.

This cholesterol-like compound is found in plant foods like pumpkin seeds. A review of four studies found it significantly improves the stop-and-go traffic of urinary flow, so you can empty out completely during your first trip to the loo.

You may get similar benefits from pumpkin seed oil. It can be pricey, but studies show it too can help urinary woes. Culinary experts suggest you use it in its raw form, rather than heated, to preserve nutrients. Try it whisked into vinaigrettes, drizzled over bread, or mixed into smoothies.

> Pumpkin seeds are often called pepitas, but are they the same thing? Technically, yes. But the culinary world uses the term pepita for the hulled, green inner seed, while pumpkin seeds include the beige outer shell. Certain pumpkin varieties actually grow the shell-less seeds.

Manly mineral shrinks your prostate. The walnut-size prostate gland houses more zinc than most other organs. And for a good reason — the mineral is essential to prostate health. Experts say zinc may reduce the size of the prostate, relieving bothersome symptoms naturally.

Make sure you get the recommended 15 milligrams (mg) of zinc daily. An ounce of hulled pumpkin seeds will give you 2.1 mg. That's 14 percent of the amount of zinc you need each day, all packed into a crunchy little snack.

Quinoa

Wheat-free way to get great grain benefits

The Incas called it the "mother of all grains," but quinoa isn't a grain at all. It's actually the seed of a plant related to spinach and Swiss chard. Even so, people still consider it the star of grains. Perhaps it's because this seed makes a great alternative for folks who can't stomach other grains.

Tease your taste buds with gluten-free fare. As exotic as quinoa (pronounced keen-wa) sounds, you can easily find it in your local grocery store, often in the rice section. It comes in three main colors — white, red, and black. These colorful seeds make a delicious side dish, quick salad topping, or healthy soup thickener. The nutty flavor pairs with a fluffy texture that's both creamy and crunchy.

Beyond its delightful taste, quinoa has another perk — it is gluten-free. People who have gluten sensitivities — or the full-blown disorder called celiac disease — react to gluten proteins found in wheat, barley, and rye with symptoms such as:

- bloating
- diarrhea
- headaches
- mood changes
- joint pain
- abdominal pain
- constipation
- skin problems
- fatigue

Perfect flour for gluten-free goodies

Going without gluten doesn't mean you have to kiss your favorite baked goods goodbye. These days you have glorious gluten-free options, including one especially nutritious surprise — quinoa flour.

You can substitute equal parts quinoa flour for all-purpose flour, but you may end up with bread or cookies that are more grainy or crumbly than you'd like. Try combining it with other gluten-free flours to see what works best.

Some folks think quinoa flour has a sour, bitter taste. Experts say you can fix this by toasting it. Spread the flour on foil, and bake at 215 degrees for 2 1/2 to 3 hours.

If you have a high-powered food processor or blender, feel free to make your own flour from toasted quinoa. Then store it in the freezer when you're done. It will be ready and waiting for your next delicious gluten-free recipe.

Go against the grain for symptom relief. Hold your horses — your doctor said you weren't gluten sensitive. But you still experience headaches, joint pain, and eczema flare-ups after eating wheat, barley, and rye. What gives?

A recent study published in *Gastroenterology* revealed wheat contains other proteins besides gluten that could cause similar symptoms or make gluten sensitivity worse. And, like gluten, they're linked to inflammation and chronic conditions like multiple sclerosis, inflammatory bowel disease, and rheumatoid arthritis.

Is quinoa a solution for these folks too? Well, an older study suggested a possible link between certain varieties of quinoa and reactions in gluten-sensitive people. So researchers created a new study to put quinoa to the test. They asked a small group of people with celiac disease to add quinoa to their diets for six weeks. Quinoa didn't make symptoms worse, passing the test with flying colors.

The one mineral you need to dodge the dangers of diabetes

Magnesium is the ninth most common element in the universe. But if you have diabetes, your body still might not be getting enough. Enter quinoa. This magnesium-rich food tackles symptoms linked to diabetes, so you can avoid dangerous health setbacks.

Mineral helps your body use sugar better. High blood sugar is the hallmark of diabetes. And it's the reason some folks with diabetes need frequent bathroom breaks. Your body can't absorb all that sugar from your blood, so the leftovers end up in your urine where it draws more water, making you "gotta go." You end up flushing a lot of nutrients — particularly magnesium — right down the toilet, leading to deficiencies.

Low magnesium levels deal a bad blow for your blood sugar. But a cup of quinoa gives you an extra boost with almost a third of the amount you need each day.

Experts say magnesium can improve insulin sensitivity, which regulates your blood sugar — even if you don't have diabetes. That breaks the cycle and allows your body to use sugar the way it's supposed to — for energy. This mineral goes the extra mile and actually helps during exercise, increasing strength and stamina.

Takes the pressure off diabetes-related health problems.
About eight out of 10 people with type 2 diabetes have high
blood pressure. But if you're in a stew about high BP, worry no
more with this little food. Again, the magnesium in quinoa is
the hero of the day.

To prove it, researchers analyzed 34 studies with more than 2,000
participants. They learned magnesium supplements lowered both
systolic and diastolic blood pressure.

- Magnesium stimulates compounds like nitric oxide that
  relax blood vessels, which improves blood flow and lowers
  blood pressure.

- It acts as an antioxidant, protecting blood vessels from
  damage caused by oxidative stress.

The participants took an average of 368 milligrams of magnesium
a day, which is close to the amount recommended for older adults.
You can easily get that much in your diet, especially if you include
quinoa and nuts like almonds, pistachios, and peanuts.

Lower blood pressure doesn't just make your doctor happy. It
also slashes your risk of complications and death related to diabetes, such as diabetic retinopathy and kidney disease.

Quinoa combos boost energy all day long

Tired and sluggish? Quinoa has a history of providing vim and
vigor. It goes way back to the Incas who ate mixtures of quinoa
and fat, called war balls, to sustain their armies as they marched
over the Andes Mountains. If fat doesn't sound appealing, you'll
be glad to hear healthier, yummier foods pair well with quinoa
to give you more energy.

Transform breakfast to energy with B vitamins. Sure, food gives you stamina. But how does your body convert that grub into power? With the help of nutrients like B vitamins. It's no surprise then that deficiencies can cause fatigue and weakness.

Luckily, quinoa has plenty of B vitamins to go around. It's particularly high in folate, with 19 percent of your daily requirements per cup. You'll also score thiamine, riboflavin, B6, and niacin. So start your morning off right with a yummy quinoa combo.

Quinoa for breakfast? Yep. It tastes great with bananas, which are also loaded with B vitamins. Warm up quinoa, stir in almond milk, a mashed banana, and cinnamon. Then sprinkle pecans on top.

> Quinoa comes in three main varieties. White, the most common type, has the lightest texture and makes a great substitute for rice. Black has a sweeter, earthier taste. Red is nuttier and holds its shape best after cooking, making it perfect for salads. It also has the most antioxidants.

Iron out common causes of fatigue. Some people know it as "tired blood," others as anemia. But no matter what you call it, the signs are the same — fatigue, dizziness, and even headaches. The most common cause is low iron levels.

Your body needs iron to make hemoglobin, a protein that carries oxygen from your lungs to the rest of your body. Without that oxygen delivery, your cells don't get the nourishment they need.

A cup of quinoa has 15 percent of the iron your body requires every day. Infuse your lunch with energy by serving up a side dish of quinoa and iron-rich cooked spinach.

Extend energy with a protein-packed meal. It takes your body longer to break down protein into usable amino acids than it does to break down carbohydrates. That means protein can give you energy longer.

Good thing quinoa rises above the rest in the protein department. A cup is loaded with 8.1 grams or 16 percent of the protein you need each day. More importantly, it contains all the essential amino acids your body can't make on its own.

To boost your energy even more, eat quinoa with protein-packed lentils. This duo takes about the same amount of time to make, so you can serve up a hot, healthy dinner in a jiffy.

Cut cholesterol with quinoa (plus 4 more ways it does your body good!)

The United Nations officially kicked off the quinoa craze when it named 2013 the International Year of Quinoa. How did this tiny food get a whole year to its name? It has a remarkable nutrient lineup that rivals other grains, even when it comes to fiber.

This roughage is what makes quinoa the perfect companion to a cholesterol-lowering diet. Plus, add it to your meals, and you'll stumble upon other fiber-driven perks.

To test the effects of quinoa on factors like cholesterol, researchers asked a small group of women to add one of two cereals to their diets. One group ate corn flakes — a fairly low source of fiber — while the other had quinoa flakes.

After a month, total cholesterol and bad LDL cholesterol went down in only the quinoa group. How does fiber work its magic? It binds with cholesterol in your gut, flushing it out of your system before your body can absorb it.

But don't think you have to go out and search for quinoa flakes to score the benefits. One cup of regular quinoa has 21 percent of the fiber you need each day. Check out four more fiber benefits you'll get from this fabulous grain.

- **Protects your heart.** The more fiber you eat, the lower your chances of heart disease and stroke.

- **Sheds the pounds.** Fiber fills you up and keeps you fuller longer.

- **Improves internal plumbing.** Foods with fiber keep things moving along and feed good gut bacteria.

- **Steadies sugar levels.** Fiber slows sugar absorption, so your blood sugar doesn't spike. It may even lower your risk of developing type 2 diabetes.

Secrets to cooking perfect quinoa

"I tried quinoa years ago," says Lauren Reagan. "I wanted to like it, but something was off about the taste." If you, like Lauren, have eaten bitter quinoa, you may have made the classic mistake of not rinsing before cooking. These days, quinoa is often pre-washed to get rid of saponins, the bitter coating that protects the seeds from pests. But some experts still say rinsing through a mesh sieve is a good idea. Here are two ways to cook up a tasty dish.

- Boil. Quinoa cooks like rice in about 15 minutes. Pro tip — don't stir quinoa with a spoon. Fluff with a fork if you want to avoid a mushy meal.

- Toast. After you rinse the raw quinoa, sauté it in a pan, stirring it around as it cooks. The wet seeds will start to pop when they begin drying out, and will turn brown when ready. It's crunch time.

Raisins

Chow down on nature's candy to win the blood pressure battle

Sugary, sweet snacks may be your guilty pleasure, but they aren't doing your heart any favors. Junk food is loaded with refined sugar, sodium, and other chemicals that jeopardize your health. Fortunately, raisins can satisfy your sweet tooth — and help you manage your blood pressure to boot.

In a recent study, researchers asked people with slightly higher than normal blood pressure to eat either raisins or prepackaged snack foods for 12 weeks. By the end of the study, people who ate snack foods saw no change in their blood pressure. But raisin eaters dropped their systolic blood pressure by as much as 10 points.

"It is often stated as a known fact that raisins lower blood pressure. But we could not find much objective evidence in the medical literature to support such a claim," says the study's lead researcher Harold Bays, MD. "However, our study suggests if you have a choice between eating raisins or other snacks like crackers and chocolate chip cookies, you may be better off snacking on raisins at least with respect to blood pressure."

Researchers couldn't pinpoint exactly why raisins were so effective, but they think it has something to do with all the potassium in these little treats. Potassium plays a huge role in controlling your blood pressure by helping your kidneys flush out extra sodium so it's not hanging out in your bloodstream wreaking havoc.

Just a single handful of raisins contains well over 200 milligrams of this critical mineral. As an added bonus, the fiber and antioxidants in raisins help relax your blood vessels so your blood flows more easily.

"Raisins are packed with potassium, which is known to lower blood pressure," Bays says. "They are also a good source of antioxidant dietary fiber that may favorably alter the biochemistry of blood vessels, causing them to be less stiff, which in turn, may reduce blood pressure."

Who knew such a tiny snack could have such a big impact?

Mythbuster: naturally sweet treats won't rot your teeth

How many times have you heard that sticky, sweet foods are enemies of your teeth? If you want to avoid cavities, raisins are probably one of the first foods you'll drop from your diet. But contrary to popular belief, raisins won't attack your teeth. Instead, they'll help you fight off cavities and keep your dentist at bay.

Cavities develop when bacteria in your mouth convert sugars from food into acid that eats away at your tooth enamel. But the natural sugar in raisins isn't the same as the sugar in candy and other sweets that bacteria like to feed on.

And even though raisins feel sticky, they don't stay on your teeth longer than most other foods. Plus they have antioxidants that attack the bacteria lurking in your mouth and keep them from digging holes in your beautiful teeth.

'Grape' way to fight off these 5 deadly diseases

Raisins are just dried grapes, so you may be tempted to think of them as the same food. But if you make that mistake, you'll be missing out on one of nature's most powerful disease fighters — resveratrol. Raisins are almost always made from green grapes, which lack this nutrient. So if you're looking to combat high blood pressure, cholesterol, diabetes, and dementia, freshen up your diet with red grapes.

Crush your risk of colon cancer. In a recent study published in *Nutrition Journal,* researchers examined the potential effects of resveratrol on colon cancer in a group of 30 healthy people. First, scientists had people eat a low-resveratrol diet for two weeks — avoiding foods like grapes, peanuts, or dark chocolate. After that, they were divided into three groups, and for the next two weeks ate either 1/3 pound, 2/3 pound, or 1 pound of grapes each day.

During the study, each person was checked for the early markers of colon cancer. Those in the group who ate more grapes showed fewer warning signs of cancer. Researchers think the resveratrol in grapes blocks the chemical messengers responsible for the growth of cancerous spots in your colon. Plus people in the study lost weight, which could have also lowered their cancer risk.

High blood pressure? High doses of resveratrol can help clear it up. Researchers from China compared six studies on resveratrol and blood pressure to see if they could measure how well the nutrient lowered BP. Turns out it's very effective at lowering systolic blood pressure — but only at high doses.

One way resveratrol may work is by keeping your body from producing hormones that drive up blood pressure. As an added benefit, it raises your production of nitric oxide, which loosens up arteries and gets your blood flowing.

The magic number where resveratrol starts helping is 150 milligrams per day. A cup of red grapes only gives you a little over 1 milligram, so you'd need to supplement to reap the benefits. Be sure to talk to your doctor before taking high amounts of resveratrol, especially if you take blood pressure medicine.

Eat your heart out — combatting cholesterol starts in your stomach. Is the way to your heart truly through your stomach? Scientists say yes. If you want to take care of your ticker, you'll have to start by looking after your gut. More specifically, you'll need to focus on the trillions of bacteria living inside your digestive tract. This community of bacteria, known as your microbiome, holds an important key to stopping atherosclerosis, commonly known as hardening of the arteries.

> Systolic blood pressure — the top number of your reading — measures the amount of pressure on your artery walls when your heart beats. The higher it is, the harder your heart is working to pump blood through your body. Keeping it low is one of the best ways to lower your risk of heart disease.

When you eat meat or other animal proteins, your gut makes a compound known as trimethylamine N-oxide (TMAO). This compound is bad news. It boosts inflammation, which creates more damage in your arteries and makes it easier for cholesterol to attach and form plaque. And if your TMAO levels get too high, your body has to work extra hard to get rid of your dangerous LDL cholesterol.

But resveratrol might hold the secret to switching this chemical off. In a recent animal study, researchers found this nutrient lowers TMAO in the blood. They think resveratrol works by keeping your microbiome from producing trimethylamine, which your liver uses to create TMAO. This still hasn't been tested on humans, but the early results are promising. Keep your ear to the ground for future updates.

Grape nutrient helps you win the blood sugar battle. In one study, 70 people with type 2 diabetes took 1,000 milligrams of resveratrol for 45 days, By the end of the study, they showed better fasting glucose and insulin levels than people using a placebo.

Scientists think resveratrol helps activate the proteins in your body in charge of signaling insulin to absorb and use sugar. They found it lowered fasting glucose and insulin levels and improved blood-sugar control and insulin sensitivity.

The amount used in the study is a huge dose, so don't try high-dose supplements without talking to a doctor first.

Sip from the fountain of youth by drinking this fruit juice. A glass of red grape juice won't actually make you younger, but it can keep your brain youthful by staving off Alzheimer's and dementia. Grape juice has a good amount of resveratrol, which can help keep your brain in tiptop shape.

Recent research conducted by scientists at the Georgetown University Medical Center found this nutrient works by literally shielding your brain from dangerous irritants.

Resveratrol boosts the power of your blood-brain barrier that keeps harmful inflammation-causing molecules from getting into your brain.

Raisin' the bar — make these tiny treats yourself

You don't have to buy your raisins by the box. Skip the expense and make them yourself. Homemade raisins can take your salad, trail mix, or midday snack to the next level. All you need is a baking sheet and an oven.

- Preheat your oven to about 225-250 degrees.

- Grab a few bunches of your favorite grapes, and remove them from the stems. Go for green grapes for a tarter treat or red grapes if you want to satisfy your sweet tooth.

- Lightly oil a baking sheet and cover with the grapes.

- Bake for three to four hours, until shriveled and dry.

- Let them cool, and enjoy. Leftovers will last about three weeks in an airtight container in the fridge.

Crank up your energy without crashing your blood sugar

A quick, sweet snack that boosts your energy and helps you dodge diabetes sounds like something created in a sports science lab. But actually it's one of the world's oldest foods — raisins.

Research has found these tiny sun-dried grapes are packed with energy-building nutrients and fiber and are an excellent choice for a pre-workout snack.

- A recent study had runners eat raisins or high-tech endurance bars while they worked out, and raisins performed just as well at keeping people's energy levels up.

- A second study found raisins actually trumped energy bars when it came to controlling blood sugar and insulin levels.

Fiber may be the secret when it comes to blood-sugar control. Raisins are chock-full of fiber, and studies show it helps improve glucose and insulin levels. That's important when it comes to fighting off diabetes. If you eat a lot of fiber, research says you're 29 percent less likely to get this disease than your friends who eat very little. A cup of raisins supplies 6 grams of fiber — about a quarter of what you need each day.

Eating raisins throughout the day is an easy way to munch your way through that cupful. Sprinkle a few on your morning oatmeal, toss some into your lunchtime salad, then grab a handful for an afternoon snack. You'll crank up your energy while keeping your blood sugar stable.

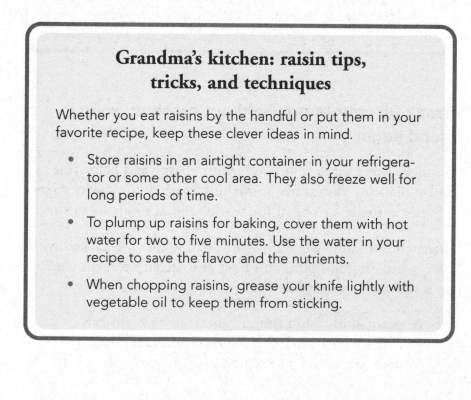

Grandma's kitchen: raisin tips, tricks, and techniques

Whether you eat raisins by the handful or put them in your favorite recipe, keep these clever ideas in mind.

- Store raisins in an airtight container in your refrigerator or some other cool area. They also freeze well for long periods of time.

- To plump up raisins for baking, cover them with hot water for two to five minutes. Use the water in your recipe to save the flavor and the nutrients.

- When chopping raisins, grease your knife lightly with vegetable oil to keep them from sticking.

Rooibos tea

3 heart-healthy secrets in every cup

The Cederberg region of South Africa. A place of towering mountains, purple sunsets, and rooibos (pronounced ROY-boss) tea. If you haven't yet sipped this rich, sweetly nutty brew, you're missing out on not only a tasty drink, but a whopper of a health boost.

The rooibos tea plant (*Aspalathus linearis*) is also called the red bush plant, because the shrub has red stems, and the fermented leaves and their tea are a bright orange-red color.

The people of South Africa began harvesting and steeping the leaves over 300 years ago, but only in the last century has rooibos tea been exported around the world. Despite efforts to grow it in other countries, today the rooibos plant still only thrives in the very specific soil and climate of Cederberg.

Fortunately, you can find rooibos tea in your local supermarket or online. And you'll want to add it to your shopping cart because:

- it is rich in natural plant compounds called polyphenols. These act as antioxidants in your body to fight damaging free radicals related to heart disease, cancer, and other health conditions. Some you may have heard of before, like quercetin and luteolin.

- it is the source of two little-known but strong antioxidants — aspalathin, which is unique to rooibos, and nothofagin.

- it is naturally caffeine-free, which means it hasn't gone through a decaffeination process that destroys polyphenols.

- it is low in tannins, so it doesn't have the drying, bitter taste of many teas.

Ready to let the nutrients in rooibos tea fight the ravages of heart disease?

Get stroke protection in place now. Damage to your brain following a stroke can be catastrophic. In fact, you lose as many vital nerve cells in your brain, called neurons, after a stroke as you do in about three-and-a-half years of normal aging. However, a recent animal study found drinking rooibos tea for seven weeks prior to a stroke protected these neurons.

Your brain is shielded by a layer of cells called the blood brain barrier (BBB). It prevents harmful substances from crossing into your brain from your general circulatory system. Experts suggest the polyphenols in rooibos tea, especially aspalathin and nothofagin, reinforce your BBB, protecting you from stroke damage caused by free radicals and inflammation.

In addition, lab studies show aspalathin and nothofagin help stop your blood from forming dangerous clots, the leading cause of thrombotic strokes.

Every cup of rooibos tea you drink now could protect you from devastation in the future.

Daily tea drinkers improve cholesterol. The *Journal of Ethnopharmacology* published a small but important study highlighting another way rooibos tea can safeguard your heart.

Forty people at risk of heart disease drank six cups of rooibos tea every day for six weeks. Their harmful LDL cholesterol levels dropped 15 percent, and their good HDL levels increased 33 percent.

Put a damper on dangerous inflammation. You may not realize it, but your blood vessels can become inflamed. It's often your body's way of responding when you're overweight, not active enough, or have too much sugar in your blood. This inflammation plays a major role in a condition called athero-sclerosis, hardening and narrowing of the blood vessels that carry blood away from your heart.

Aspalathin and nothofa-gin in rooibos tea are proven to control this inflammation, again by working as antioxidants in your body.

> Green rooibos tea is brewed from the plant's unfermented leaves. While it has a lighter color than the fermented red rooibos tea, it tastes a bit like regular green tea. More importantly, green rooibos has more antioxi-dants than red since the process of fermentation destroys some of these healthy compounds.

Rock-solid bones are just a teacup away

Rooibos tea has unique properties that make it especially valu-able for maintaining a strong skeleton. While it contains many nutrients that nurture bone growth, it also fights osteoporosis in two delicious ways.

- Most teas contain natural chemicals, called polyphenols, that boost your bones' important minerals — calcium, phosphorus, magnesium, and potassium. Two in particular, luteolin and orientin, are in rooibos tea, and were recently studied at Brock University in Canada. Researchers there found these polyphenols improved mineral levels in bone-building cells called osteoblasts.

- The National Osteoporosis Foundation reminds you to limit caffeine, since it decreases the amount of calcium you absorb. The good news — rooibos tea is naturally decaffeinated. That makes it a smart alternative to other teas that have to go through a chemical process to remove the caffeine.

> ## Best brew news: it's always teatime
>
> There's no real mystery to brewing a perfect cup of rooibos tea. The best advice is to take your time. By steeping your leaves for at least 10 minutes, you'll get a beautiful deep red tea brimming with a boatload of antioxidants.
>
> Most people find rooibos has a smoother, sweeter taste than other teas, probably because it contains few of the usual drying compounds called tannins. But feel free to add milk, honey, or lemon to taste. None will affect the health benefits.
>
> You may want to brew a whole pot of this calming beverage at once, and keep some for later. No worries. Either enjoy an icy glass straight from the fridge or reheat a cup in the microwave. No bitter taste here.

Stop your toxic response to stress

Hormones are powerful. As chemical messengers, they affect how you grow, how your body works, and how you feel. A tiny imbalance can have serious repercussions.

Take cortisol, for instance. It's the hormone your adrenal glands release whenever your brain reacts to stress. It triggers a burst of sugar in your blood for energy, tells your brain to use that glucose, and encourages tissue repair.

Too much stress over a period of time, though, means too much cortisol. And that can make you feel anxious or depressed, bring on headaches or sleep problems, cause you to gain weight, and even play a part in developing heart disease.

People who drink rooibos tea report feeling calmer, but scientists were never sure why. Now they've discovered the natural compounds in rooibos — including aspalathin and nothofagin — help control the amount of cortisol your adrenal glands produce.

Sardines

Bone up with this dynamic duo

Under the sea, under the sea, darling it's better down where it's wetter, take it from me ...

These lyrics from Disney's *The Little Mermaid* ring true when it comes to the benefits you'll find swimming around in the ocean. Even the tiniest fish, like the sardine, packs a nutritional punch.

One of sardine's most surprising contributions to your diet? Calcium. A 3.75-ounce can of these little fish contains 351 milligrams — more calcium than a glass of skim milk. It's a great way to help make sure you get the recommended 1,000 to 1,200 milligrams a day.

Your skeleton is a bit like a nutritional piggy bank, storing up calcium and other minerals. If you skimp on calcium, your body takes it from your bones to use wherever it's needed. That can lead to osteoporosis and possibly a broken bone.

Fortunately, your body is great at rebuilding your skeleton as long as you keep giving it the right fuel. And that means more than just calcium. Vitamin D is critical, too, because it helps your body absorb calcium from foods.

Lucky for you, these tiny fish are a super source of vitamin D as well as calcium. You'll get more than 60 percent of your daily dose of D from eating a small can of sardines. Try them on crackers with a dash of sour cream or yogurt for a quick and nutritious snack or light lunch.

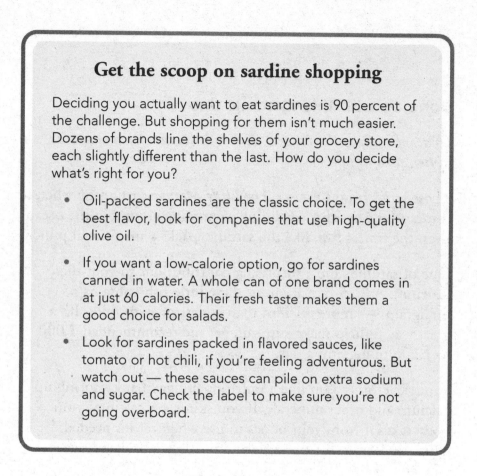

Get the scoop on sardine shopping

Deciding you actually want to eat sardines is 90 percent of the challenge. But shopping for them isn't much easier. Dozens of brands line the shelves of your grocery store, each slightly different than the last. How do you decide what's right for you?

- Oil-packed sardines are the classic choice. To get the best flavor, look for companies that use high-quality olive oil.

- If you want a low-calorie option, go for sardines canned in water. A whole can of one brand comes in at just 60 calories. Their fresh taste makes them a good choice for salads.

- Look for sardines packed in flavored sauces, like tomato or hot chili, if you're feeling adventurous. But watch out — these sauces can pile on extra sodium and sugar. Check the label to make sure you're not going overboard.

Beyond brittle bones — 4 ways calcium can surprise you

Calcium is a surefire way to ward off weak bones, but that's not all this common mineral is good for. It can fight forgetfulness, high blood pressure, poor digestion, and even some cancers, too. So don't let osteoporosis take center stage — this mineral deserves the spotlight in any conversation about what ails you.

Can't remember where you put your keys? Call on calcium.
Keeping your calcium levels up is an important part of staying
sharp. The mineral boosts the levels of important chemical messengers, like dopamine, in your brain. And if your calcium levels
are low, you're at a higher risk for mental decline as you age.

Shore up your defenses against high blood pressure.
Studies have been up and down about how well calcium helps
with blood pressure. But many have shown an inverse relationship, meaning the more you have in your body, the lower your
blood pressure.

Scientists think calcium helps stabilize the cell membranes in
your blood vessel walls, which relaxes the arteries. It works with
sodium, potassium, and magnesium to provide this balance and
keep your blood pressure in check.

If you're worried about sardines being too salty, this should make
you feel better. Experts say higher calcium levels may offset the
effects of salt on your blood pressure.

Calcium — a boon to poor digestion. If you're dealing with
digestive woes, try adding more calcium to your diet. It plays a
big role in helping you absorb nutrients from your food.

One more weapon to fight off cancer. Calcium for colon
cancer? Maybe so. In a recent review of studies, researchers
found that for every 300 milligrams of calcium you eat each
day, your risk of colon cancer goes down by 8 percent. Adding
a can of sardines to your daily menu would do the trick.

Experts think one way calcium protects your intestines is by
binding with bile acids and fatty acids to create compounds
called calcium soaps. Just like regular soap protects your skin
from germs, these soaps protect the cells lining your colon from

damage. And if those cells start multiplying, calcium helps keep them in check.

Another recent study produced good news about calcium and ovarian cancer. Researchers focused on African-American women because they've shown a high risk of dying from this disease. They also tend to be low in calcium and vitamin D. The scientists found that eating a high-calcium, low-lactose diet may reduce the women's risk for this type of cancer.

Memory trouble? Vitamin B12 will banish your forgetfulness

Keeping your body in tiptop shape is impossible without a healthy diet. The same goes for your mind. If you want to fight off dementia, Alzheimer's disease, or fading memories, you need to get the right fuel.

And vitamin B12 is nature's high-octane gas when it comes to your brain. This vitamin tunes up an area called the hippocampus, which is where your long-term memories are formed and stored. But you may hit a little bump in the road — as you get older, your body has trouble absorbing enough of this essential nutrient.

You need to fight back by tracking down foods rich in vitamin B12. And guess which little fish is overflowing with this particular vitamin? That's right, sardines. A single can gives you all the vitamin B12 you need for the day, plus a third of the next day's.

You may think you're getting enough B12 in your diet, but don't take any chances. A recent study shows that if your levels are on the low side of normal, your memory may still suffer.

Don't pass up this finn-tastic source of vitamin D

Lounging in the sun is the perfect way to spend a summer day. While it may seem like you're not doing anything, your body is hard at work producing vitamin D. You make this nutrient just by soaking up sunlight. How easy is that? But here's the catch. As you get older, your body has a harder time doing it successfully.

That's why you should focus on eating vitamin D-rich foods like sardines. You need 600 international units (IU) of vitamin D every day, 800 IU if you're over 70. A small can of sardines gets you most of the way there by providing 63 percent of your daily requirement.

Vitamin D keeps heart disease at bay. That's what scientists found when they analyzed 34 heart-related studies. They saw an inverse relationship between vitamin D and heart disease. That means the more vitamin D in your body, the less likely you'll have heart problems. And if you don't get enough, you open yourself up to serious conditions like high blood pressure, which can lead to heart attack and stroke.

> Your tuna sandwich may taste good, but it may also be loaded with mercury. This dangerous metal builds up in large fish, so if you opt for small fish like sardines, you'll dodge harmful toxins. Because sardines grow quickly, pollutants don't have time to store up.

So grab a can of sardines and strike back. Vitamin D works overtime to protect your blood vessels from damage. Plus it helps keep your blood pressure from getting out of control.

Chicken soup for your cold? Try sardines, instead. Gulping down orange juice while eating a steaming pot of chicken noodle soup is one way to keep infections away. But if you're skimping on sardines, you're missing out on some prime protection.

British researchers analyzed 10,000 people and discovered vitamin D can help thwart respiratory infections. This amazing nutrient actually pumps up your immune system and wards off dangerous germs.

The amount varied from study to study, but don't worry about going a bit overboard. You can safely get around 4,000 IU of vitamin D a day.

The sunshine vitamin melts away the pounds. Are you having trouble shedding that spare tire? You might need to add a little vitamin D to your diet. New research claims if you're overweight and low on vitamin D, supplements may help you lose those extra pounds.

Scientists in Italy looked at overweight and obese people who were deficient in vitamin D. They compared groups taking monthly doses of 25,000 IU or 100,000 IU of vitamin D to those taking no supplement. After six months, guess who lost more weight and inches from their waistlines? Way to go, vitamin D.

How does it work? Studies show this powerful vitamin may help prevent fat from forming. Evidence also suggests vitamin D may improve insulin sensitivity, which could lead to weight loss.

Sea vegetables

Seaweed — a 'shore' thing for weight loss

Seaweeds, or sea vegetables, are a lot like the plants that grow in your garden — only they grow in water. Oh, and they may just be the perfect food for health and weight loss. They contain all the essential minerals and trace elements your body needs. Plus, they're low in calories but rich in fiber, vitamins, and healthy fats.

If you're thinking "eeewww," you're probably thinking of raw seaweed, which can feel slimy. You don't have to eat it that way. You can fry it, steam it, and even eat it dried like potato chips.

Take your pick. Sea vegetables come in three varieties — red, brown, and green. Most have exotic-sounding Japanese names like wakame and nori. The Japanese have been enjoying these plants since at least 600 B.C., but lots of cultures eat them. Thanks to online shopping, health food stores, and the spread of Asian supermarkets, even landlocked people can get them.

Super fiber blocks your body from absorbing fat. Some sea veggies are supercharged with fiber. Take these three. Ounce for ounce, they pack more fiber than brown rice or bananas.

- sea spaghetti (officially known as *Himanthalia elongata*), a brown seaweed you can cook and eat like pasta

- dulse (*Palmaria palmata*), a red one you can fry like bacon

- kombu (*Laminaria digitata*), a brown one used to flavor soups

Alginate, a special fiber in these plants, could block your body from absorbing up to 75 percent of the fat you eat. That could cut your fat intake and your calories. Alginate blocks an enzyme that your body uses to digest fat. If you can't break it down, you can't absorb it, so it passes out of your body.

That's exactly how Orlistat, a prescription weight-loss drug, works. Unfortunately, Orlistat can cause serious side effects. Experts think sea vegetables can do the same thing more safely. This fiber may also help you feel fuller after eating, which could help you eat less and lose weight. If you're looking to stay slim, why not give seaweed a try?

> Can't stand seaweed? You can buy Xanthigen, a supplement that contains fucoxanthin. Obese women who took 600 milligrams of Xanthigen daily lost weight and body fat, plus shrunk their waistlines. But remember, you'll miss out on the fiber and other compounds that make seaweed so healthy.

Want to shed more pounds? Check out fucoxanthin. This funny-sounding antioxidant, found mainly in brown seaweeds, may help you shed unwanted fat. Studies show it shrinks body fat, lowers triglycerides, and boosts "good" HDL cholesterol. It may work even better if you eat it with other healthy compounds, like:

- conjugated linoleic acid (CLA). This combination was better at keeping animals from gaining weight. CLA is found mostly in grass-fed meats and dairy products.

- fish oil. Eating fucoxanthin with this oil helped keep animals from gaining fat. Try eating salmon with a side of cooked sea spaghetti.

New wonder food whisks away toxins

Forget colon cleanses and detox diets. Eating sea vegetables may cleanse cancer-causing toxins like dioxin from your body naturally.

Dioxins are highly toxic pollutants that end up in the foods you eat, particularly meat, dairy, fish, and shellfish. They can cause cancer, harm your immune system, and mess with your hormones. And they're tough to get rid of. They build up in your liver and fat cells and can linger in your body for years, even decades.

That's where brown sea veggies, like wakame and kombu, may help. Research shows the fiber and chlorophyll in these seaweeds provide a one-two punch against dioxins. Not only do they block your cells from absorbing them, they help flush dioxins out of your body faster. That means less bad stuff building up in your body.

Sea veggies turn the tide on diabetes

Brown sea vegetables are loaded with compounds that could help you avoid diabetes, slow it down if you have it, and even ward off deadly complications like heart attacks. Drug companies are desperately trying to turn these natural compounds into high-priced drugs. You don't have to wait for that. Get these sugar-busting benefits easier and cheaper by eating the food itself.

Go brown to dial down diabetes. It may not be your favorite color, but it's the one to pick to keep your blood sugar on an even keel. Brown sea vegetables like wakame and sea spaghetti are the sole sources of two special compounds that could prevent diabetes.

- fucoxanthin, an antioxidant that helps your cells absorb and use glucose

- phlorotannins, which seem to protect the pancreas cells that make insulin

As the disease creeps up on you, the extra sugar in your blood gradually kills these pancreas cells, leading to full-blown diabetes. Together, these two compounds form a dynamic duo that could stop that from happening.

Help your blood sugar stay in check. When your liver pumps out more glucose than your body can use, you wind up with high fasting blood sugar. Phlorotannins could help control this, too. A specific one called dieckol tells your liver to dial back the glucose, which in turn could lower your fasting blood sugar.

Seaweeds put a lid on after-meal sugar spikes. Topping your next meal with mekabu or a side of toasted nori may save your life someday. Seriously. Blood sugar can rise quickly after a meal, and research shows a direct link between after-meal spikes and your risk of stroke, heart attack, and other types of blood vessel blocks.

Healthy adults who ate white rice — known to send blood sugar skyrocketing — had a much smaller spike if they ate a brown seaweed called mekabu with it. Nori, a red seaweed, had the same effect. People's blood sugar spikes were one-third lower if they ate a single sheet of dried nori with their meal.

> You can buy mekabu dried and packaged. Follow the directions for soaking it. Then add it to your omelet as you would spinach, or use it to garnish pasta and other grains. Nori comes in dried sheets. Toast them lightly on each side, and munch on them in place of potato chips.

Both types of seaweed are full of gel-like fiber, similar to oatmeal. That may slow down your digestion so you absorb the sugar from food more gradually.

Or maybe you can thank those phlorotannins again. They block you from digesting carbohydrates and breaking them down. If you can't break them down into glucose, then your blood sugar won't shoot up after you eat.

Either way, your body benefits.

Flu fighters from the sea

Next winter, give yourself a better shot at avoiding the flu. Eat some seaweed. *Undaria pinnatifida*, which wakame and mekabu come from, is rich in fucoidan, a compound that fights inflammation and possibly viruses.

Seniors who ate fucoidan sprinkled on their lunches every day had more virus-fighting immune cells than seniors who didn't eat seaweed sprinkles. They also had a stronger immune reaction to the flu shot. That's a good thing. It means the vaccine worked better and made them less likely to catch the flu.

Flu vaccines don't protect you as well when you're older because your immune system weakens with age. Goose yours into higher gear by eating a quarter cup of seaweed salad made from wakame, or a small side of mekabu. You can also buy granules made from brown seaweeds and use them in place of table salt.

2 reasons not to go overboard on seaweed

Sea vegetables are great sources of sodium and iodine. Sometimes too great. Eat them sparingly if you're on a low-sodium diet, or choose varieties that tend to have less salt. Rinse them before use to further cut the salt.

Lowest in sodium	Highest in sodium
nori (*Porphyra umbilicalis*)	Irish moss (*Chondrus crispus*)
dulse (*Palmaria palmata*)	egg wrack (*Ascophyllum nodosum*)
sea grass (*Ulva intenstinalis*)	wakame (*Undaria pinnatifida*)

A little iodine can benefit your thyroid, but too much can harm it. If you've had thyroid problems in the past, talk to your doctor before adding sea vegetables to your diet. Large amounts of iodine can cause thyroid problems even if you've never had an issue before.

Lowest in iodine	Highest in iodine
nori (*Porphyra umbilicalis*)	sea grass (*Ulva intenstinalis*)
sea lettuce (*Ulva lactuca*)	kombu (*Laminaria digitata*)
Irish moss (*Chondrus crispus*)	egg wrack (*Ascophyllum nodosum*)

Most people handle the extra iodine in sea vegetables just fine. But contact your doctor right away if you develop symptoms like anxiety, insomnia, shaking hands, and racing heart, or forgetfulness, depression, and constipation.

Tainted seaweed: a tsunami waiting to happen

Sea vegetables soak up whatever is in the water around them, the same way land vegetables absorb what's in the soil. If the water is polluted with heavy metals — say lead, arsenic, mercury, or cadmium — seaweeds may absorb them. Eating them can raise your risk for cancer and other health issues.

Stay safe. Vary the kinds of seaweeds you eat as well as the brands. Make sure the company selling them screens for toxins. And avoid the seaweed called hijiki *(Hizikia fusiformis)* and any supplements made from it. It tends to have high levels of inorganic arsenic, the most toxic kind.

Sea plants turn your garden green

The next time you're at the beach, take a look at the fresh seaweed washed up onto the shore. No, you can't take this home and eat it, but organic gardeners know it's a great way to feed your soil.

Seaweed, or kelp, provides some of the main three minerals plants need — nitrogen, phosphorus, and potassium — along with other trace elements like magnesium and zinc. You can add it to your compost pile, or chop it up into your garden bed before you put in new plants. Along with adding nutrients to the soil, seaweed also helps ward off slugs.

Follow local rules for gathering seaweed from commercial beaches. Then take it home and rinse it well before you use it to remove excess salt.

Spinach

Spinach: a nutrient-filled feast for your eyes

A rainbow on the horizon. Clear starry nights. A breathtaking sunrise. Ralph Waldo Emerson put it beautifully when he wrote, "The sky is the daily bread of the eyes."

But your eyes can't live by bread alone. They need specific nutrients to keep your eyesight sharp for years. Make leafy greens — like spinach — a star on your salad bar, and your vision will never fade to black.

Fight eye disease and keep that twinkle in your eye. Spinach and other leafy greens are rich in lutein and zeaxanthin, two plant compounds called carotenoids. This sight-saving duo protects your eyes from dangers like pollution and the sun's ultraviolet rays. Sort of like all-natural sunglasses built right into your eyes.

These important nutrients also make up the pigment in your eye's macula, the part of the retina responsible for sharp central vision. The macula is tiny, roughly the diameter of a pencil eraser, but it's critical to helping you see clearly. Without it, you couldn't make out the details of objects in front of you, like your morning paper or needlepoint.

That's the type of problem you'll experience if you develop age-related macular degeneration (AMD). Your macula will start to thin and break down, and eventually you'll notice things are off with your vision. Straight lines may seem bent, or you may have difficulty recognizing faces. As the disease progresses, a blurred spot forms in the middle of your field of vision, making it difficult to read, write — even drive.

Experts don't know what actually causes AMD, but some of the risk factors include age, family history, smoking, exposure to bright sunlight, environmental pollutants, and obesity.

Spinach can help save your sight. A healthy diet can't cure AMD, but it can help slow its progress. Some experts recommend you take up to 30 milligrams (mg) of a lutein supplement every day. But don't rush off to the health foods store just yet. You can easily get that much lutein and zeaxanthin in your diet. Just one cup of cooked spinach gives you an eye-popping 20 mg of the two carotenoids your eyes crave.

So pile your plate with green superfoods like kale, turnip greens, Swiss chard, collard greens — and of course, spinach — to keep AMD at bay. A healthy choice that's easy on the eyes.

Drizzle on a little dressing to wring all the nutrition out of your salad greens. It's easier for your system to absorb leafy green's lutein if it's combined with a fat like soybean oil, found in most salad dressings. Limit your serving, though. Just 32 grams — about two tablespoons — will do the trick.

This power couple can KO high blood pressure

If Popeye and Curious George packed their favorite foods in your lunch box, you'd head off to work with more than just a delicious meal. The magnesium in Popeye's spinach paired with the potassium in George's bananas make a healthy combination that can do wonders for your blood pressure.

Drop your pressure with this popular pair. Turns out potassium and magnesium are quite the nutritional duo. Everybody knows bananas are packed with potassium, right? But did you know one of potassium's main jobs is to relax the walls of the blood vessels? And that helps lower your blood pressure.

> Steer clear of limp veggies. To keep your spinach and other produce fresh, simply place a clean, dry sponge in the refrigerator drawer with them. The sponge will absorb excess moisture, so your fruit and vegetables will stay fresh for days — or even weeks — longer. An easy and economical tip.

But once you finish off George's favorite fruit, how does the potassium get where it needs to go? That's where its partner, magnesium, comes in. Found in dark leafy greens like spinach, whole grains, beans, and nuts, magnesium regulates many body systems, including blood sugar, muscle function, and energy production. But magnesium is also responsible for moving potassium into cells, where it can help balance sodium levels — crucial for healthy blood pressure.

A tasty way to boost your magnesium. The National Institutes of Health reports most older adults don't get the right amount of magnesium. Low levels of the mineral can lead to nausea, sleepiness, and weakness. But experts warn getting too much magnesium — like with a supplement — may cause diarrhea and stomach cramps. To be sure you get the right amount, just make good food choices.

For example, you can pump up your lunchtime sandwich with a layer of bright green spinach. Toss a handful of chopped fresh spinach into your spaghetti sauce or canned soup. Simply adding a cup of the cooked greens to your dinner menu will boost your magnesium intake to around 157 milligrams (mg). That's about half the recommended daily amount for women — 310 to 320 mg — and almost 40 percent of the 400 to 420 mg suggested for men.

Nothing wimpy about that.

Cook your greens to brush off spinach tooth

That gritty film covering your teeth after you eat spinach actually has a name. It's called "spinach tooth," and it's caused by a plant chemical — oxalic acid — found in spinach.

When you chew the leafy greens, the oxalic acid combines with the calcium in spinach, forming calcium oxalate crystals that float around in your mouth. And that's spinach tooth.

Your body normally eliminates these crystals through the stool or urine. But, in some people, the crystals may end up in the kidneys, raising the likelihood that kidney stones will develop.

Love spinach but don't want to risk kidney stones? Boil or steam your veggie to get rid of the oxalic acid. Prefer a fresh spinach salad? Squeeze some lemon juice over the raw greens. The ascorbic acid — vitamin C — in the lemon juice will dissolve the oxalic acid.

Prostate cancer protection from a humble leaf

Hip, hip, hooray! Three cheers for spinach. This humble veggie is so packed with key nutrients, just two servings each week is enough to measurably reduce the risk of developing aggressive prostate cancer.

Experts know spinach is chock-full of healthy nutrients like beta carotene, lutein, and zeaxanthin, just to name a few. But one compound found in this popular vegetable actually causes prostate cancer cells to self-destruct. It's called neoxanthin.

Spinach beats back cancer cells. In one Japanese study, researchers discovered the neoxanthin in spinach killed three types of the human prostate cancer cells they tested, including nearly 100 percent of the cells associated with lymph node carcinoma of the prostate (LNCaP). The other two types of cancer cells tested, PC-3 and DU 145, also showed significant decreases. Pretty impressive.

Another study, this one in Canada, backed up the health benefits of the spinach leaf. After studying almost 30,000 men for four years, experts found more than 1,300 had developed prostate cancer. But the men who ate the most veggies — like broccoli, cauliflower, and spinach — were less likely to see their cancer progress to a life-threatening stage than those who rarely ate them.

Pile on the greens for prostate protection. Good news for spinach eaters. When it came to this leafy green, the men in the study who ate more than two cups a week benefited the most. They showed a lower risk of developing the aggressive form of prostate cancer than men who ate less than one serving a month.

Do you prefer your spinach sautéed with garlic or fresh off the salad bar? Doesn't matter, say the researchers. You can reap the benefits of neoxanthin no matter how you eat it. But remember — not even a superfood can keep you cancer-free. Your best defense? Aim for a healthy, balanced diet, packed with at least five servings of fruits and vegetables every day.

How to make sure your greens are clean

The Dirty Dozen. No fruit or vegetable wants to make this list. But unfortunately for spinach, it recently clinched the Environmental Working Group's No. 2 spot, right behind strawberries. According to researchers, the conventionally grown spinach samples they tested had twice as much pesticide residue as any other crop.

A report from the U.S. Department of Agriculture showed 75 percent of spinach samples contained permethrin, a neurotoxic insecticide. At high doses, permethrin — banned in Europe — may damage the nervous system, causing tremors and seizures. It's even been linked to attention deficit hyperactivity disorder (ADHD) in children.

Thoroughly rinsing your spinach leaves under running water may help get rid of some of the pesticides. But you can avoid these dangerous chemicals altogether by purchasing organically grown produce. To be sure your spinach is organic, look for a 9 at the beginning of the Price Look Up (PLU) number on the produce label.

Strawberries

Better off red — 3 sweet ways to treat your ticker

Native Americans called ruby red strawberries "heart-seed berries." But it's not just their shape and vivid color that bring your ticker to mind. Experts say strawberries are good for your heart in more ways than one. And it all comes down to their bold hue.

Lay out a bunch of berries, and you'll see they have something in common — deep rich colors. Notice the bold red of straw-berries and raspberries. Check out the dark blues and purples of blueberries. What you see are anthocyanins. And they're not just pigments. They're also health-boosting nutrients that act as antioxidants to boost three aspects of your heart health.

Cut cholesterol with the raw power of berries. Anthocyanins and other antioxidants are the heavy hitters behind balanced cholesterol levels. They block free radicals from damaging blood cells and making cholesterol more dangerous.

To see if the antioxidant powers of strawberries could help lower cholesterol, researchers put it to the test. They asked vol-unteers to eat about three cups of fresh strawberries daily. After a month, bad LDL cholesterol went down almost 14 percent.

Give high blood pressure a red light. High BP causes the walls of your blood vessels to narrow, reducing blood flow and making your heart work harder. Anthocyanins help boost blood flow, so your heart can take a break.

One study looked at 14 years of data on more than 155,000 people from three big studies. Researchers found that participants who ate the most food containing anthocyanins — mostly from blueberries and strawberries — had an 8 percent lower risk for high BP.

Bag cleaner berries with one scrumptious strategy

Every year, the Environmental Working Group — an organization dedicated to protecting the health of people and the environment — ranks the fruits and vegetables most likely to be contaminated with pesticide residues. What food scored number one out of all the Dirty Dozen? You guessed it — strawberries.

So how do you gain the juicy benefits of strawberries without the dangers of pesticides? Go organic. That doesn't mean you have to spend more at the grocery store. Try growing your own strawberries. Experts say it's easier than you may think.

You don't have to have a big garden. You just need a small space and plenty of sun. Strawberries also grow well in pots or hanging baskets. Plus, they're perennials, so they'll keep producing succulent berries for about five years.

Ask your local nursery or garden center which variety will work best for you.

Colorful berries ax your risk for heart attack. The scariest part of heart glitches is you often have no clue there's a problem until you're propped up in a hospital bed after a heart attack.

But eating strawberries may help lower your risk of heart attack, says a long-term study of more than 94,000 women.

The research, published in the American Heart Association's journal *Circulation*, focused on foods containing anthocyanins. Over 18 years, women who ate more than three servings a week of strawberries and blueberries cut their risk of heart attack by a third compared to those who ate them once a month or less.

"We have shown that even at an early age, eating more of these fruits may reduce risk of a heart attack later in life," says lead author Aedin Cassidy, Ph.D.

Don't think of strawberries as just for dessert. Try adding them to pancakes, cereals, salads, and smoothies for a delicious and healthful boost to your meals.

'Berried' treasures bump up brain power

Madame Tallien, a royal who lived during the rule of Emperor Napoleon, once bathed in the juice of 22 pounds of fresh strawberries. While that sounds like a delicious dip in the tub, here's a better use for all those berries. Add them to your plate for a snack that's jam-packed with brain benefits.

And you don't have to eat 22 pounds a day. Snacking on a cup or more of strawberries or at least one half-cup of blueberries each week could do the trick, says a study published in *Annals of Neurology*.

These berries are the top contributors of anthocyanins and other flavonoids. The nutrients give berries their color and come with other health benefits — like protecting from mental decline by boosting your memory and thinking ability.

Do berries really make a difference? To find out, researchers used data from more than 16,000 women in the prestigious Nurses' Health Study. The results showed brain aging could be delayed by up to two-and-a-half years in older women who ate greater amounts of the flavonoid-rich berries.

Experts point to two ways berries boost brainpower.

- All those antioxidants safeguard your cells from vandalism caused by hazardous free radicals.

- Berry nutrients also support your brain's nerve cells by fighting inflammation. This protects against damage that can affect motor control, memory, and thinking skills.

Savory and saucy — 2 unexpected ways to dish out strawberries

Berries and dessert go together like strawberries and shortcake. But sometimes you want a healthier sweet treat. Try this — blend berries with yogurt and spread a thin layer in the dehydrator for a nutrition-packed fruit roll-up. Then test out two more fresh ways to devour strawberries.

Make it savory. Strawberry recipes don't have to be sweet. Picture them with onions, mozzarella, and spinach. It may sound like a strange combo, but it tastes heavenly on a pizza. Or skip all the work and pile ricotta or goat cheese, basil, and strawberry slices on crackers for a quick snack.

Serve it up saucy. Spice up any dish with a tasty dressing. Simply blend strawberries with balsamic vinegar and olive oil. Depending on what you have a taste for, you can add more ingredients. Want a spread for your chicken dinner? Add garlic, pepper, and your favorite spices. Rather keep it simple? Just pour over a salad.

Snack on strawberries to support your waistline

Crackers, candy, and chips, oh my. All three made the list of the most popular snack foods in America. But if you want to stay trim, you'll have to swap out these fattening foods for a more wholesome choice. Check out three science-backed nutrients that make strawberries a delicious alternative.

Flavonoids. You'll find these plant compounds in fruits like strawberries, blueberries, grapes, and pears. If you eat a lot of these foods, you may have less weight gain over time.

That's what researchers found in a recent 24-year study published in *BMJ*. They reviewed data from 124,086 participants in three long-running health studies and found some encouraging results. Flavonoids may lower the amount of fat your cells absorb, increase the number of calories you use throughout the day, and block the formation of fat.

Vitamin C. People who don't get enough vitamin C may be more resistant to fat loss, says a study. But get the right amount of vitamin C, and you could burn 30 percent more fat during exercise than folks with low vitamin levels. That's because vitamin C has a hand in exercise performance, stamina, and fat burning.

Did you know your body absorbs iron better when you eat iron-rich grub with food filled with vitamin C? Soak it all in with strawberries. Ounce for ounce, strawberries have more vitamin C than oranges.

Good news — a cup of sliced strawberries has 163 percent of the vitamin C you need each day.

Fiber. And don't forget to bulk up — with fiber. That same cup of strawberries has 13 percent of the fiber you need daily. A recent study showed that a high-fiber diet helps with weight loss.

Roughage fills you up, so snacking on strawberries will make you feel full longer and keep you from nibbling on other things.

Pick cancer-killing berries for a burst of flavonoids

Want a head start on cancer prevention? Strawberries are the first fruits to ripen in the spring. Add in their track record for crimping cancer, and you have a yummy first defense against the big C.

Strawberries get their kick from a powerhouse of flavonoids. These plant compounds are the stars of a recent study published in the *American Journal of Clinical Nutrition.* Researchers recruited more than 1,000 women over the age of 75 and followed them for five years. They recorded 73 percent fewer cancer deaths in ladies who ate the most flavonoids compared to those who ate the least.

What strawberry flavonoids rock the park? Anthocyanins and flavonols like fisetin, kaempferol, and quercetin show up in research again and again. They may lower your risk for esophageal, ovarian, bone, colon, and bladder cancers. That's one mouthwatering benefit of eating more strawberries.

But how does it work? Well, flavonoids do a number on cancer cells in more ways than one.

- Oxidative stress caused by free radicals can trigger inflammation and damage to your cells and DNA. Berry nutrients protect your body by going after the free radicals before they do any damage.

- These cancer-fighting nutrients also stop the growth and spread of dangerous cells by aiding in apoptosis, a process your body uses to destroy unwanted cells.

Sweet potatoes

Perfect way to perk up your memory

Candied, whipped, grilled, or baked, there's no doubt about it. Sweet potatoes are one of the most nutritious veggies you can eat. Why wait 'til Thanksgiving to gobble them up? Tap into this tasty root any time you're looking to nourish body and mind.

Sweet potatoes provide a big bang for the buck. Low in calories and with no fat or cholesterol, sweet potatoes are packed with digestion-promoting fiber and roughly 25 percent more potassium than bananas. They're also a great source of the mineral manganese, which your body needs to burn carbohydrates and fat as well as absorb calcium and regulate blood sugar.

Sweet potatoes are chock-full of beta carotene, the pigment that gives fruits and vegetables their vibrant yellow and orange colors. Your body converts beta carotene into vitamin A, a necessary nutrient for healthy skin, laser-sharp vision, and a strong immune system. One medium-sized, baked sweet potato provides more than four times the amount of vitamin A you need in a day. But don't worry about wasting all that extra nutrition. Your liver stores excess vitamin A for when you're running low.

Lost your slippers? Slip in some antioxidants. It turns out the beta carotene in sweet potatoes has an added benefit. It's a powerful antioxidant that may help prevent memory loss.

Researchers at Brigham and Women's Hospital and Harvard University discovered this after following 6,000 men age 65 and older as part of the long-term Physicians' Health Study II. Those taking beta carotene supplements for 15 years or more performed better on mental tests, including the ability to remember things. But those who took the supplements for three years or less showed no gains. Scientists think even slight improvements in memory can make a big difference in your risk of developing dementia.

The researchers in the Physicians' study believe beta carotene's antioxidant power helps improve communication signaling between neurons in the brain. It also appears to make the brain more resistant to toxic beta-amyloid proteins, which form the plaques found in the brains of people with Alzheimer's.

Rooting out the differences in yams and sweet potatoes

Popeye famously declared, "I yam what I yam." Truth be told, he may have mistaken the yam for a sweet potato. Many do, even though the two veggies are unrelated.

Sweet potatoes were first cultivated thousands of years ago in Latin America. Their skins range from cream to red, yellow, purple, and brown. You'll recognize them by their pointed ends.

Yams are bullet-shaped and have dark, bark-like skin. Most come from Africa and can grow up to five feet long. Yams are drier and starchier than sweet potatoes and have a slightly nutty taste.

Why the confusion? It's thought that slaves in the Americas called the sweet potato "yam" because it reminded them of the food they ate in Africa. The name stuck, particularly in the American South.

Beware too much of a good thing. You may want to think twice about beta carotene supplements if you're a smoker. Studies show high-dose supplements may significantly increase your risk of lung cancer. They can also interact with prescription medications.

The men in the study benefiting from the extra beta carotene took just 50 milligrams every other day. That's about the same amount you'll find in two cups of baked sweet potatoes. To be on the safe side, health care professionals recommend you get your beta carotene from a healthy diet that features lots of antioxidant-rich fruits and vegetables.

Toss back 'taters to juice up your joints

Swollen, painful joints? Stiff in the hips? Fortunately, sweet potatoes' antioxidant powers don't stop at memory loss.

This super spud may also slow the progression of osteoarthritis (OA), a painful disease that occurs when cartilage, the spongy tissue that covers your bones, wears away. Risk factors for OA include injury, joint stress from being overweight, and getting older.

So how can antioxidants halt OA in its tracks? It comes down to chemistry. When your body converts oxygen into energy, it often produces too many "free radicals" that damage cells. In the case of OA, the unstable compounds target already weakened cartilage tissue. Experts think antioxidants such as beta carotene neutralize the free radicals and make them harmless.

Boston researchers put this idea to the test. In a long-term study of adults with OA in their knees, those who took in more than 9,000 IU of beta carotene a day were less likely to see their arthritis worsen than people who got less than 5,000 IU. Plus they also ran a lower risk of experiencing severe knee pain in the future.

According to the U.S. Food and Drug Administration, most people only get about 3,300 IU of beta carotene a day. Want a super simple way to triple that number? All you have to do is eat half a baked sweet potato to get the beneficial amount used in the study. A whole medium sweet potato will provide a whopping 21,907 IU of this powerful antioxidant.

Sweet or white? A handy primer on potatoes

A potato is not a potato is not a potato. But you know that. You grab tiny, new red ones for an elegant chive-topped side dish. Yukon Golds are great for mashing. And when it comes to a stellar baked potato, nothing beats the classic Russet. The Potato Association of America — yes, it exists — recognizes 92 varieties, including a blue potato. But wait, we aren't even talking about sweet potatoes yet.

Around the world, you'll find thousands of varieties of this sugary spud, but you're most likely to see the Beauregard and Jewel at your local supermarket. Because they grow best in warm, sunny climates, sweet potatoes used to appear on menus and kitchen tables only in the South. But once the rest of the country got up to speed on this nutritional powerhouse, you began to find sweet potato lovers in every ZIP code.

Of course, all kinds of potatoes are naturally low in fat, sodium, and cholesterol, but you'll find white and sweet shine in different areas.

Check out this quick comparison of nutrients for 200 grams of potato. That translates into about a 7-ounce potato or one cup of canned sweet potato.

	Baked sweet potato	Canned sweet potato	Baked white potato
Calories	180	216	186
Fiber	6.6 g*	6.0 g	3.0 g
Sugar	13 g	11.4 g	3.4 g
Beta carotene	23,016 mcg***	11,002 mcg	0
Converts to vitamin A	769% Daily Value	367% Daily Value	0
Vitamin C	39.2 mg**	21.6 mg	25.6 mg
Vitamin E	1.4 mg	2.4 mg	0
Vitamin K	4.6 mcg	5.2 mcg	0.6 mcg
Iron	1.4 mg	1.8 mg	0.8 mg
Potassium	950 mg	386 mg	782 mg

*grams (g)   **milligrams (mg)   ***micrograms (mcg)

Sweet (and healthy) way to take a bite out of diabetes

Weighing in at just 180 calories per cup, sweet potatoes' health-boosting benefits keep growing. So much so, that the American Diabetes Association (ADA) has placed the nutrient-dense veggie on its list of the top 10 diabetes superfoods.

Stamp out sugar spikes. That's because sweet potatoes, despite being a starchy vegetable, have a surprisingly low glycemic index. They release sugar into your bloodstream at a steady and slow pace, helping you to avoid sudden spikes in blood sugar. In fact, the ADA says people with diabetes should substitute sweet potatoes for white potatoes, which have a higher glycemic index.

High fiber gets a high five. One cup of mashed sweet potatoes has more than 8 grams of fiber, a whopping one-third of the recommended daily amount. All that fiber keeps you feeling full longer and less likely to snack. That's a good thing since overweight people carry a greater risk of developing type 2 diabetes, the most common form of the disease.

Fiber also seems to keep blood sugar in check. That's according to Texas researchers, who asked more than a dozen adults with type 2 diabetes to follow two diets over separate six-week periods. One of the diets featured 50 grams of fiber, the other had a more moderate 24 grams.

> Boiled sweet potatoes have half the glycemic index of baked or roasted, making them a better choice for people with diabetes. Along with helping you avoid blood sugar spikes, boiling makes it easier for your body to absorb all the nutrients that sweet potatoes have to offer.

The results? Blood sugar levels fell significantly when participants were on the high-fiber diet. The scientists aren't sure why but say one reason may be that fiber reduces or delays the body's ability to absorb carbohydrates.

Follow Japan's lead for better blood sugar. The Japanese have treated diabetes with white sweet potatoes for hundreds of years. A research team at the University of Vienna tested the Asian folk remedy by giving men with type 2 diabetes either sugar pills or low or high doses of white sweet potato powder. The men took the pills three times a day over six weeks. Sure enough, those who took the high doses became less resistant to insulin, and their blood sugar and cholesterol levels dropped.

Treat yourself royally with purple potatoes

The land of luaus, volcanos, and Don Ho is also home to a little-known root — the Hawaiian purple sweet potato. Whether sliced for chips or whipped into a pie filling, this eye-catching edible is a healthy addition to any menu.

Hawaiian sweet potatoes get their rich purple shade from anthocyanins, the same compounds that give color to blueberries, eggplant, and red cabbage. They act as antioxidants that, researchers say, lower the risk of heart disease and stroke in people with high blood pressure.

You can buy purple sweet potatoes, dubbed "uala" in Hawaii, over the internet and at specialty markets. It's best to store these vibrant veggies in a cool, dry place, where they'll remain fresh for a week or two. Then swap them out for the more traditional orange-fleshed variety in your favorite recipes. Try roasting them with butter and cinnamon, or mashing them for a colorful side dish that brightens up your table.

Tofu

Learn to love soy to crack down on cancer

Tofu is the enemy of meat-lovers everywhere. After all, who hasn't seen a good burger or turkey ruined by this pale, flavorless substitute? But there's a reason people have been eating this nutritional powerhouse for more than 2,000 years. It's loaded with protein, calcium, and other great nutrients. Better yet, tofu can help you ward off two of the most common cancers.

The myth about soy and breast cancer. You may be avoiding tofu and other soy-based products because you've heard it raises your risk for breast cancer. For years doctors thought this was true. This idea was based on a study that showed a naturally occurring phytoestrogen in soy can switch on cancer-causing genes — in mice.

But people and rodents don't process soy the same way. New studies say you don't have anything to worry about. And if you do get diagnosed with breast cancer, you may actually want to start eating more soy.

New findings — soy helps you beat breast cancer. Scientists recently analyzed five studies involving more than 11,000 women with breast cancer. They found the women who ate more soy foods like tofu were less likely to have their cancer recur. And those who ate the most soy lived longer, too.

Researchers think soy works by binding with chemical receptors in your cells that are normally reserved for estrogen. This keeps too much estrogen from getting into your cells, which is good because estrogen helps breast tumors grow.

Studies show soy isoflavones start protecting you from breast cancer in childhood. And the longer you eat soy, the stronger your protection. That doesn't mean it's ever too late to start. Research says women who don't eat much soy in their youth actually gain more protective benefits from soy products like tofu later in life.

Take the mystery out of tofu

Convincing your family to add tofu to the dinner table is only half the battle — shopping for it is a daunting challenge, too. Here's how to find the perfect package of tofu for any occasion.

Tofu is sold by firmness, which describes how much water has been pressed out of it. Each has a slightly different flavor and texture, so experiment with different kinds to find your favorite.

- Silken or soft tofu. These tofus are smooth and soft. They can be blended into sauces, smoothies, and even used as a dairy substitute when baking.

- Medium tofu is the all-purpose choice. It can work in almost any recipe that calls for tofu, and it's great simmered in soups or baked.

- Firm tofu is the toughest of the bunch, so it won't fall apart when it's cooked. Try it in stir-fries or curries.

Soy isn't just for women — this powerhouse can protect your prostate. Men, don't skimp on soy foods either, even if you do prefer meat. Studies of Asian populations suggest men who eat the most soy-based foods are half as likely to get prostate cancer. Believe it or not, tofu's estrogen-blocking powers may work the same way for men as for women. Researchers think soy isoflavones bind to the estrogen receptors in the prostate and block the growth and spread of tumors.

While you may not like tofu burgers or tofurkey sandwiches, don't give up on this healthy food. It's delicious in Asian-inspired salads, stir-fries, and curries.

Bone up on soy to block osteoporosis

You may not know it, but you just broke a bone. Don't worry, your bones are actually designed to break a tiny bit at a time. They store important minerals and nutrients for your body, but the only way to get them out is to slowly break them down and build them back up. It's an easy process as long as your body gets the right fuel — and tofu is one of the best bone-builders you can find.

Crank up the calcium to protect your skeleton. Calcium helps keep your bones strong, so you need a lot of it in your diet. If you run low, you're at risk for brittle bones.

Tofu is a lot like cheese. It's made from soy milk that has been curdled and pressed into blocks. And just like dairy, tofu is a great source of calcium. A half-cup serving contains almost half your daily recommended dose. If you want even more bang for your buck, look for brands that use calcium sulfate. This traditional ingredient used to curdle soy milk boosts the mineral content of tofu.

Soy blocks your bones from breaking down. Women are hit hardest by osteoporosis because menopause causes you to produce less estrogen. This hormone helps your body hang on to calcium, so low levels put you at risk for osteoporosis. Some doctors prescribe hormone treatments or drugs to stave off bone loss, but these procedures can be risky. Fortunately, tofu boasts a natural solution.

Soybeans are loaded with natural chemicals, called isoflavones, which are remarkably similar to estrogen. Research published in the *American Journal of Clinical Nutrition* found isoflavones keep your bones from breaking down too quickly. They work by tricking your body into thinking it's getting a natural hormone and helping you hold on to calcium.

Isoflavones are key to slowing bone loss. When compared to conventional osteoporosis drugs, isoflavones fall a bit short — but they come without any of the nasty side effects. And other research seems to back this up. A study at the University of Hull in the United Kingdom also found that taking moderate doses of isoflavones slowed down osteoporosis in postmenopausal women.

"We found that soy protein and isoflavones are a safe and effective option for improving bone health in women during early menopause," says lead author Thozhukat Sathyapalan. "The actions of soy appear to mimic that of conventional osteoporosis drugs."

The women in the study got around 66 milligrams of isoflavones a day. That's a lot for most Americans but not for the typical Asian diet. One 3-ounce serving of tofu has 19 milligrams of soy isoflavones, so that's a good place to start.

Snacking on tofu won't weigh you down

A morning of hard work and careful dieting goes down the drain when you open a bag of potato chips to soothe an afternoon craving. But skip the snack and you'll overeat at dinner. Try snacking on tofu instead — it will fill you up and help you lose weight at the same time.

Eat more protein to tip the scales in your favor. A recent study published in *The Journal of Nutrition* revealed tofu might just be the perfect afternoon snack. This high-protein wonder food can help you gain control of your appetite.

Researchers asked a group of teens to eat either a high-protein snack, a fatty snack, or no snack at all in the afternoon. After four days of testing, they discovered the teens who ate the protein-rich snacks were less hungry and showed better appetite control throughout the rest of the day.

The young people in the study ate a soy-based pudding. The high-protein version clocked in at 25 grams of protein. You can get about 10 grams from a half-cup serving of tofu.

If you want an easy afternoon snack, try baking your tofu. Just toss sliced, firm tofu in oil, and bake on a parchment-lined sheet in a 400-degree oven. Take it out after about 25 minutes or when golden brown. This crispy treat will satisfy all your afternoon cravings.

Natural soy chemicals block fat from forming. Filling your stomach with protein isn't the only way soy can help you shed a few pounds. Researchers think soy's isoflavones can actually battle fat, too. Estrogen is a fat-storing hormone. Isoflavones are so similar to estrogen, they bind with chemical receptors in your cells meant for estrogen. This blocks your cells from storing fat.

Estrogen also plays a big role in fat distribution. Low estrogen levels produce deep belly fat, which is more harmful than fat located just under the skin. Eating soy with isoflavones that mimic estrogen tricks your body into redistributing the fatty tissue away from your belly, where it's easier to lose.

The trouble with too much tofu

You're tossing tofu into your stir-fries and salads, drinking soy milk, and snacking on roasted soy nuts. But now you wonder — is there such a thing as too much soy?

When it comes to stroke risk, the answer may be yes. A large study recently found that Chinese women who ate the most soy had a small but significant increase in their risk of stroke. Turns out soy isoflavones, which are plant estrogens, may cause the same problems in post-menopausal women as hormone therapy.

The top soy eaters in the study took in roughly 60 milligrams of isoflavones a day. You'd have to eat about a half pound of tofu — two-thirds of a block — to get that much from food. But if you're combining it with other soy products, you could easily go over.

If you'd like to eat more soy-based foods or take an isoflavone supplement, talk with your doctor to assess the risks.

Turmeric

Worried about cancer? 8 great reasons to try turmeric

"Let food be thy medicine and medicine be thy food." Wise words from the ancient Greek physician, Hippocrates, who lived nearly 400 years before the birth of Christ. Perhaps the "Father of Medicine" was referring to turmeric, a savory spice from southern Asia that had found its place among popular medicines thousands of years before he was born.

Turmeric's active ingredient, curcumin, is a powerful antioxidant that protects the body from molecules known as free radicals. They can weaken your cell's membranes, damage the DNA, and even cause cell death. But turmeric has other super-powers besides blocking nasty free radicals.

Scientists have found this "queen of spice" may help prevent and treat eight types of cancer. Adding just a quarter teaspoon to your menu every day may be just what the doctor ordered to fight off these deadly diseases.

Breast cancer. Studies have shown curcumin can slow the spread of cancer cells, increase cell death, and prevent angiogenesis, the development of new blood vessels that support cancerous tumors.

Colon cancer. A study at Kingston University in Great Britain tested selected herbs and spices, including turmeric, bay leaf, ginger, and sage. The spices, especially turmeric, were found to block the growth of human colon cancer cells, also known as HCA-7. And researchers at the Anderson Cancer Center in Texas also discovered fresh turmeric root may be even more effective in fighting colon and other types of cancer cells than curcumin alone.

Head and neck cancer. A team of researchers discovered curcumin blocked head and neck cancer cell growth by binding with an enzyme known as IKK. But in order for the turmeric to fight this cancer, experts say it must be taken in supplement form because the amount needed is much higher than what is normally used in cooking. In the study, participants took two supplements totaling 1,000 milligrams daily.

Leukemia. Combining curcumin with green tea's EGCG was found to increase the apoptotic — cell death — process in chronic lymphocytic leukemia. The treatment worked best when people took EGCG first followed by the curcumin.

Lung cancer. About 85 percent of diagnosed lung cancer is non-small-cell lung cancer (NSCLC). According to some studies, turmeric's curcumin may slow the development and progression of NSCLC by blocking cancerous A549 cells from invading other tissue.

Melanoma. One study found curcumin caused apoptosis, a programmed cell death, in melanoma, the most dangerous form of skin cancer.

Beware. In some cases, turmeric may do more harm than good. Turns out it can lower the anti-tumor action of some chemotherapy drugs. And some studies show curcumin can be harmful if you're on blood-thinning therapy. Best advice? Talk to your doctor before adding turmeric to your health plan.

Pancreatic cancer. In one small study, curcumin was shown to slow the growth of this deadly cancer. And participants reported no serious side effects even when they took as much as 8 grams — about one and a half teaspoons — of the spice every day. Experts suggest pairing curcumin with omega-3 fatty acids like olive oil to prevent, and even kill, pancreatic cancer cells.

Prostate cancer. According to the World Health Organization, one-third of cancer deaths could be prevented if people ate more natural compounds — like turmeric's curcumin. Which compounds are most effective against prostrate cancer? Resveratrol found in red grapes, ursolic acid in apple peels, and — you guessed it — turmeric. Researchers said combining the ursolic acid of apple peels with either turmeric or red grapes blocked the prostate cancer cells from getting glutamine, a nutrient necessary for their growth.

Turmeric is a perennial plant that grows five to six feet high in the tropical regions of southern Asia — especially India, the world's largest producer. The plant roots, also called rhizomes, are boiled, dried and ground, turning them into the bright orange-yellow powder that gives curry and other Asian dishes their special flavor.

Golden spice keeps you in the pink

Are you dreading the health problems that seem to come with old age? You know the ones. Osteoporosis, heart disease, Alzheimer's, osteoarthritis. You've already read about turmeric's cancer-fighting power. Now read on to find out how this one spice can help treat and prevent those age-related diseases, too.

Heart disease. Atherosclerosis, a big word for a big problem. You may know it better as hardening of the arteries. This

condition develops when fatty deposits called plaque —
made up of cholesterol, cellular waste, calcium, and a clotting
material called fibrin — clog up your arteries.

Researchers studied curcumin's effect on this disease by giving a
half gram of curcumin, a little more than a pinch, to volunteers
for seven days. The results? The researchers noted a 12 percent
drop in total cholesterol levels. And HDL — the good cholesterol — increased by 29 percent.

In another study, 14 men were fed either a meal of rice mixed
with turmeric, garlic, ginger, red pepper, and cumin or a control meal without the spices. Scientists found the spicy meal
improved after-dinner blood flow, which in turn reduced the
risk of heart-related problems.

2 easy ways to boost turmeric's benefits

Turmeric can do your body good — as long as it gets a little
help from a couple of culinary cohorts. First, add a little
healthy fat. Your body has trouble absorbing turmeric
properly. In fact, as soon as you get some in, your liver tries
to get it out. And if you can't absorb it, curcumin can't do
its job. Give your body a fighting chance by cooking up
your turmeric with a good-for-you fat, like olive oil.

Next, sprinkle on a pinch of pepper. Black pepper contains
piperine, a compound that keeps curcumin from breaking
down in your liver and digestive system too quickly. And
the longer curcumin can stay in your system, the more
benefits you'll reap. Just a quarter of a teaspoon of black
pepper increases curcumin's bioavailabilty — how easily it's
absorbed by your body — by 2,000 percent.

Osteoporosis. Does the thought of holes in your bones frighten you? It should. That's what happens to your bones when you have osteoporosis. The name means "porous bone" and it's a serious condition where bones lose mass and density, making them more likely to break.

How can curcumin help? Experts believe turmeric helps build and repair bone mass. Italian researchers studied 57 people with low bone density, a condition called osteopenia. If left untreated, osteopenia can develop into osteoporosis.

In the Italian study, half the participants received a curcumin supplement along with standard treatment for osteopenia. The other half of the study group followed the standard treatment only. After six months, the supplement group saw the bone density in their finger, upper jaw, and heel increase significantly. Researchers concluded curcumin supplementation could be an important step in preventing and managing osteopenia.

Alzheimer's disease. Want to increase your chances of a life without Alzheimer's? Just eat foods loaded with turmeric. Plaques of sticky beta-amyloid protein clump together in the brains of people with Alzheimer's and worsen the development and progression of the disease.

Although research results vary, some studies suggest curcumin's anti-inflammatory and antioxidant properties change the beta-amyloid and help boost brain function while slowing the development of dementia. Experts know it's safe to take up to 4 grams per day of curcumin — about one teaspoon.

Osteoarthritis. What can you do to soothe those achy joints? Spice up your menu with a sprinkle of turmeric, or — if you don't care for turmeric's taste — add a turmeric supplement to your daily routine.

Turns out turmeric's curcumin reduces the symptoms of osteoarthritis. In fact, researchers found taking 1,000 milligrams (mg) — around a quarter teaspoon — of curcumin each day for eight to 12 weeks lessened pain and inflammation just like the NSAIDs ibuprofen and diclofenac sodium, but without the harmful side effects.

Curcumin confusion: pop a pill or sprinkle the spice?

Which is better for you? Curcumin extracts or the ground turmeric right off your kitchen spice rack?

Researchers know getting up to one teaspoon of turmeric every day has lots of health benefits. And studies show ground turmeric may have some disease-fighting compounds you won't find in extracts. But turmeric powder contains only about 3 percent curcumin, the powerhouse compound that treats illnesses like cancer and heart disease.

In turmeric extracts, the curcumin concentration may be as high as a whopping 95 percent. That means in a capsule containing just half a gram of turmeric extract — little more than a "pinch" — you could get up to 400 milligrams of curcumin.

Bottom line? If you're targeting a particular health condition, an extract may be your best choice. Otherwise, just sprinkle the spice on soups and sauces to your heart's content.

India's gold beats the blues

Caught with your hand in the cookie jar a little too often? Napping all afternoon instead of visiting friends? Forgot where you left your car keys again?

Overeating, oversleeping, and forgetfulness are just a few of the many signs of depression. This all-too-common illness can make you feel as if the whole world has lost its color, its vibrant hues turned to gray. A sprinkle of bright orange turmeric — also known as India's gold — may be just what you need to beat the blues.

Brighten your world with a simple kitchen spice. People with depression often suffer from chronic inflammation that lowers the amount of the brain chemicals dopamine and serotonin. These feel-good neurotransmitters are in charge of brain functions like mood and motivation. So if you're cheerfully cleaning out that closet you've been wanting to tackle, you can bet your levels are high. Curcumin provides a natural way to boost dopamine and serotonin so you can enjoy those positive feelings more often.

Experts have learned when you're depressed, your body also undergoes more oxidative stress. That means harmful molecules called free radicals are flooding your system, sending all the major organs in your body — including your brain — into a tailspin. Turmeric's power player, curcumin, is a natural antioxidant that can fend off those destructive free radicals and help prevent a downward spiral.

How to ditch the moody blues. In one Chinese study, scientists tested curcumin on more than 100 men suffering with depression. Volunteers were asked to take two capsules containing 1,000 milligrams (mg) of either curcumin or soybean powder every day. After six weeks, a standard depression questionnaire showed the curcumin group's symptoms improved significantly compared to the soy group.

Another study followed more than 50 people with major depressive disorder who received either 500 mg of curcumin twice each day or a placebo for eight weeks. Again, people taking curcumin felt significantly better than those on the placebo, especially after four to eight weeks.

Research is showing strong support for the brain benefits of turmeric. To help beat the blues, it can't hurt to go for the gold.

Turmeric spices up tea time

Spice up your life — and boost your health — with a warm cup of turmeric tea. Start by boiling two cups of water. Next add one teaspoon of ground, grated, or powdered turmeric. Simmer for about 10 minutes. Then strain the tea into a cup, and set it aside to cool for five minutes.

Next comes the fun part. Add the palate pleasers you prefer, maybe some lemon, lime, cinnamon, or ginger. Craving a little something sweet? Spoon in a dab of honey or maple syrup.

Don't forget to stir in some fat like whole milk, almond milk, cream, or perhaps a tablespoon of coconut oil. Then spice it up with a little black pepper. That will help your body absorb the beneficial curcumin. A delicious and healthy pot o' gold.

Vinegar

Put the brakes on 3 serious conditions

Belly fat. Diabetes. Heart disease. Definitely not your three amigos. But the older you get, the more likely you'll be dealing with one or all of them. Want to keep that day from coming? Make friends with vinegar, and you'll have a buddy who will help defend your health from problems like these. Here's how.

Vinegar can shrink belly fat. Who'd have thought a simple condiment could do what all your dieting and exercise couldn't? But it's true — Japanese researchers actually put it to the test.

The scientists divided people who were dangerously over-weight into three groups. Each group drank a 16-ounce beverage daily for 12 weeks with different amounts of apple cider vinegar — either one tablespoon, two tablespoons, or none at all.

Both vinegar groups dropped pounds and shaved inches from their muffin tops, even the group that chugged just one table-spoon a day. Experts think the acetic acid in vinegar breaks down existing fat or prevents it from forming to begin with.

Of course, you shouldn't give up exercise and eating right, but vinegar just may be that little extra something that gives you a slimmer tummy.

A little bit with your meal steadies blood sugar. Scientists across the country have been testing vinegar on people with diabetes or prediabetes for years with awesome results.

Researchers at Arizona State University found that two table-spoons of vinegar a day — one with lunch and another at dinner — improves blood sugar levels in people at high risk for diabetes. The kicker? It works even better than two leading prescriptions. They think one reason may be that acetic acid helps keep carbohydrates from being digested, and carbs can make your blood sugar spike.

Does the thought of drinking straight vinegar make you cringe? Even if it doesn't, it's not a good idea. Participants in the Arizona study drank a beverage made with 1 tablespoon apple cider vinegar, 8 ounces of water, and a pinch of sweetener immediately before meals to keep their blood sugar on an even keel. Now, that you can probably handle. Just make sure you talk with your doctor first if you take diabetes medication.

> Have you ever wondered if vinegar goes bad? Some experts say it can last indefinitely if stored in a cool, dark place like a cupboard. But for the best taste and quality, nutritionists recommend one year if opened and two years if not. That goes for all varieties.

Vinegar keeps your arteries clean as a whistle. When you shower, your body feels clean and refreshed, ready to tackle the day. Why not scrub your insides, too — with vinegar?

- If you struggle with high cholesterol, vinegar may help. Past studies have shown that the acetic acid in vinegar reduced cholesterol and triglycerides in animals. In a recent study, people with high cholesterol and triglycerides took two tablespoons of apple cider vinegar twice a day for eight weeks. Researchers found the vinegar significantly lowered these harmful fats in their blood.

- Cardiologists in Japan studied the effects of vinegar on the arteries of postmenopausal women. The women drank a 3-ounce liquid at breakfast, either with or without a tablespoon of rice vinegar added to it. Rice vinegar boosted the production of a gas called nitric oxide, which relaxes arteries and improves blood flow. Once again, researchers believe acetic acid is the magic ingredient.

- Another group of Japanese doctors studied balsamic vinegar and think it's even better for your heart than rice vinegar. Balsamic is made from grapes, which are loaded with natural compounds called polyphenols. These mighty nutrients block LDL cholesterol from causing inflammation in your arteries. Not only do you reap the benefits of vinegar's acetic acid, you get it from polyphenols, too. It's a win-win.

Problem with ants?
3 kitchen staples to the rescue!

No one wants to use dangerous pesticides in their home — and never in the kitchen. But if you have pests — especially ants — you can find nontoxic repellants right in your pantry.

- Vinegar. Tell ants to take a hike in your kitchen by washing your vinyl floor, cabinets, and laminate countertops with a mixture of vinegar and water.

- Cinnamon. Keep ants out by pouring a barrier of cinnamon along their favorite points of entry.

- Salt. Spread salt along doorways and watch ants turn around before you can say, "Shoo!"

Is vinegar the key to blocking out cancer?

Japan has one of the lowest rates of cancer in the world, and it may be in part due to vinegar.

Researchers there tested a variety of Japanese vinegars on cancer cells either in labs or on animals with promising results. Vinegar blocked the growth of colon, lung, breast, bladder, prostate, and esophageal cancers, as well as leukemia cells.

Experts think the phenolic compounds in Japanese vinegars promote antioxidant activity and neutralize free radicals. Free radicals harm cells, triggering the early stages of cancer, so anything you can do to stop the damage before it starts lowers your risk.

Fruit vinegars in particular, like sherry, balsamic, and apple cider, are chock-full of natural ingredients that fight cancer.

Stay tuned as scientists continue to research vinegar and explore its potential as a medicinal food.

Get germ-free produce in a jiff

You can't see them, but they're there — E. coli, Salmonella and other bugs — living on your apples, strawberries, and summer squash, ready to make you sick as a dog.

You don't have to worry about them any longer. It takes just two quick steps to get germ-free produce in your own kitchen.

First, grab a spray bottle and fill it with 3/4 cup water and 1/4 cup white vinegar. Then, spray your fruits and vegetables, and rinse them with tap water. Ta-da! No more bugs.

Secret to deep cleaning your home without toxic chemicals

You don't have to use chemical-filled sanitizers and fresheners when you have this amazing natural solution in your kitchen cupboard. From your bathroom to your living room, and areas in between, vinegar can clean and freshen it all.

Smart way to lower laundry costs. This common household product makes a cheap and effective substitute for many of your washing supplies. For instance, you can stop wasting hard-earned money on expensive fabric softener. Just add a quarter cup of white vinegar to your washer's final rinse cycle. Your clothes and bath towels will come out feeling soft, without soapy residue. Worried about the sour smell? No need — it goes away as your items dry.

Forget pricey stain removers, too, at least for deodorant and antiperspirant marks. Simply dab a little vinegar on the area, and wash as usual.

Say so-long to scrubbing the bathroom. Want a spotless bathroom without breaking your back? Reach for vinegar. You won't have to scrub and scrub your toilet anymore. You can just spray that ugly water ring with vinegar and walk away. Let it soak overnight, then flush in the morning. It's that simple.

For even better results, add one to two cups of vinegar to your toilet bowl before you go to bed. Flush when you get up the next day. Bye-bye waterline.

Same goes for the filmy buildup in your tub and on your shower door. Spray with vinegar, then wipe the grime away with water.

For corrosion on fixtures, dip a towel in vinegar, and wrap around faucets and shower heads overnight. Wipe clean in the morning.

Tough carpet stains are no match. When Fido has an accident, act quickly to remove tough urine stains from carpet. Here's how.

Soak up as much urine as you can with a clean rag, then dab on a solution of warm soapy water and white vinegar. Blot several times. Next, pour club soda over the spot. Blot with a clean rag until it gets soggy. Finish by applying a fresh, dry towel.

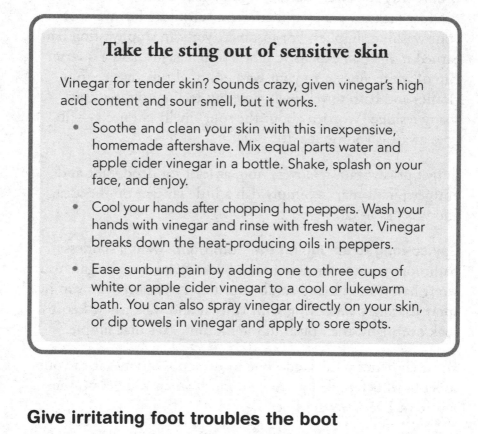

Take the sting out of sensitive skin

Vinegar for tender skin? Sounds crazy, given vinegar's high acid content and sour smell, but it works.

- Soothe and clean your skin with this inexpensive, homemade aftershave. Mix equal parts water and apple cider vinegar in a bottle. Shake, splash on your face, and enjoy.

- Cool your hands after chopping hot peppers. Wash your hands with vinegar and rinse with fresh water. Vinegar breaks down the heat-producing oils in peppers.

- Ease sunburn pain by adding one to three cups of white or apple cider vinegar to a cool or lukewarm bath. You can also spray vinegar directly on your skin, or dip towels in vinegar and apply to sore spots.

Give irritating foot troubles the boot

There's no fun in fungus, especially when it crawls all over your feet. Fight back with vinegar. It's powerful enough to disinfect your feet without damaging your nails or skin.

How to wipe out nail woes. Annie can tell you. Her fungus spread silently between her big toenail and nail bed. Since she slipped on socks and sneakers almost every morning, she didn't notice it until it was time to polish her nails for a summer party.

"I wanted to wear these cute sandals, but almost half my toenail was a yellowish color," says the Miami native. "I couldn't believe it. Even though polish would cover it, I didn't like the idea of having an infection." For months, she tried DIY remedies that didn't work. That's when she decided to do a little research.

"I read somewhere about cutting back the nail and soaking my foot in vinegar and water, so I did," says Annie. "I was supposed to do it twice a day for several weeks."

She also saw a tip about covering her toenail with Vicks VapoRub and a sock after the vinegar soaks, but she only did that once or twice. "And I got tired of doing the vinegar soak after just four or five days," she says. Still, it was enough. The nail grew back healthy, and the fungus has not come back in over 10 years.

Natural way to stomp out athlete's foot. You don't have to be an athlete to get the itchy, burning rash between your toes known as athlete's foot. All you need is exposure to conditions ripe for bacteria to thrive — wet shoes and socks, and warm, humid temperatures. Plus, athlete's foot loves to spread from person to person in places like saunas and locker rooms.

Before you try expensive medications, go the natural route. Simply soak your feet in a solution that's one part vinegar and four parts water for 10 to 15 minutes a day until the infection clears up. Bonus feature — vinegar freshens up stinky feet.

Zip up ordinary meals with these

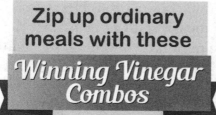

Winning Vinegar Combos

Balsamic vinegar

Fruity with hints of sweet and sour

Reduce on the stove, then pour over pork or strawberries. Can you say, "Mmm?"

Sherry vinegar

Warm and toasty

Simmer 1/2 cup vinegar with 1/2 cup brown sugar over medium heat to make a syrupy glaze. Thin with a teaspoon of water. Brush over grilled fish or chicken.

Rice vinegar

Light and slightly malty

Don't just use it in stir-fries. Drizzle over fruit or veggie side dishes like broccoli or fruit salad.

Fruit vinegar

Satisfies your sweet tooth

Combine three parts oil with one part of your favorite fruit vinegar and a bit of honey to taste. Sprinkle over grilled fruit. Make room for seconds!

Herb vinegar

Mellow goodness from your garden

Infuse 1 cup fresh basil, rosemary, or tarragon in 2 cups of a warmed, mild-tasting vinegar. Steep for three weeks then remove the herbs. Splash on salads.

Cider vinegar

Crisp and fresh

Add a teaspoon of unfiltered apple cider vinegar to a beverage that's 1/2 cup unsweetened tea and 1/2 cup apple juice. Great for fall gatherings. Even better year-round.

Wine vinegar

Rich and bright

Sprinkle on grilled mangoes and pineapples with a little olive oil and a squirt of lemon. Tastes like a tropical paradise.

Cheap and easy treatment for swimmer's ear

Don't wait to see if the pain in your ear goes away on its own. You could be asking for even more pain and swelling, or worse, a bacterial infection. That's because the water trapped in your ear canal just sits there festering, with no plans to escape. Your best bet is to treat it immediately.

Make a solution that's equal parts white vinegar and rubbing alcohol. Squirt a few drops in your ear with a baby syringe or a clean dropper, and allow the solution to drain back out.

The home remedy will zap the moisture in your ear while killing germs.

Make room for vinegar in your cold and flu survival kit

This jack-of-all-trades may help put you out of your stuffed-up, can't-breathe, throat-is-killing-me misery. Try these germ-fighting remedies the next time you're down for the count.

Surefire way to soothe a sore throat. When it hurts so badly you can't swallow, grab some vinegar and make this gargle.

- Pour 1/2 cup apple cider vinegar and 1/2 teaspoon salt into a glass jar, and set aside.

- In a separate bowl, pour 1/2 cup boiling water over 2 tablespoons dried sage or 4 tablespoons fresh.

- Cover and steep for 15 minutes.

- Strain the sage solution, and add the liquid to your jar with the salt and vinegar.

- Gargle three times a day.

- Cover your jar with a tight-fitting lid, and store in your refrigerator for up to a week.

Clear up clogged sinuses fast. Nothing feels better than breathing freely when you're sick. Relieve stuffy nasal passages with this simple addition to your vaporizer, recommended by the Vinegar Institute.

Include 1/4 cup or more of vinegar in the amount of water the unit's instructions call for. Allow the vapor to fill the room. Breathe a sigh of sweet relief.

> Here's a tip that'll make you ask, "Who knew?" Dip a cotton ball in distilled white vinegar and wipe bare nails before you apply polish. Color sticks to your nails better because the vinegar removes any natural oils that may act as a barrier. Plus, it prevents chipping. Two thumbs up.

21 surprising uses for vinegar in the kitchen

Vinegar has no substitute. What other pantry staple cleans your floors, spices up a salad, and softens kitchen towels? But wait, there's more. Check out these new ways to take advantage of vinegar's versatility.

- Wrap cheese in cheesecloth or a paper towel that's been dipped in vinegar and drained. Place in a zipper bag. It will keep mold away for longer without affecting taste.

- Wipe mixing bowls and beaters with white vinegar before whipping egg whites to remove leftover oil or grease.

- Add vinegar to the water when cooking stinky veggies like cabbage and cauliflower to keep odors at bay.

- Out of buttermilk? Add a tablespoon of vinegar to a one-cup measure, then fill the rest with regular milk.

- Get rid of pesky fruit flies with apple cider vinegar. Set out cups of vinegar on countertops. Or pour vinegar into a bowl and cover with plastic wrap. Punch holes into the plastic with a needle. Flies dive in, but can't get back out.

- Poach an egg in the microwave by cracking it in a safe dish, adding 1/3 cup of water and a teaspoon of vinegar, and cooking for a minute at 80 percent power. Continue cooking for 20 seconds at a time until it reaches poached perfection. Vinegar helps egg whites set quickly.

- Make frozen vinegar cubes and toss into a stinky garbage disposal to crush bacteria.

- Prevent sticky pasta by adding 2 teaspoons vinegar to 4 quarts water before cooking.

- Replace salt with 1/8 teaspoon vinegar in stews, soups, and sauces to tone down bitter flavors and add zest.

- Freshen up kitchen sponges and dishrags overnight by tossing them in a solution of 1/4 cup vinegar and just enough water to cover them.

- Clean the sharp edge of a rusty knife or cutting shears by pouring white vinegar over the blade and rubbing with coarse salt using a cork. Rinse with water and dry thoroughly.

- Brighten stainless steel cutlery and appliances by wiping with a cloth moistened with vinegar.

- Make a scented kitchen cleaner by adding rosemary sprigs and three lemon rinds to a solution that's equal parts water and vinegar. Avoid using on marble or granite countertops and hardwood floors.

- Sweeten your kitchen's scent by boiling water and vinegar with cinnamon and orange peels.

- Perk up wilted greens in 2 cups cold water and 1/2 teaspoon vinegar.

- Wipe away cutting-board stains caused by beets or cherries with distilled white vinegar. Just blot with a sponge, scrub, and rinse with water.

- Pour vinegar over frozen meat to tenderize it and make it thaw quicker.

- De-gunk food particles in your microwave by bringing 1/4 cup white distilled vinegar and 1 cup water to a boil. Gets rid of funky odors, too.

- Bake the flakiest pie crust ever by adding a tablespoon of chilled apple cider vinegar to your dough. Apple pie never tasted so good!

- Take the "stank" out of your lunch bag or cooler. Rinse the inside with a water and vinegar solution. If that doesn't do it, soak a towel in vinegar and place it inside overnight.

- Soak plastic ice cube trays in undiluted vinegar for four to five hours to remove hard water spots and disinfect. Rinse with cold water and dry thoroughly.

Water

1 easy way to keep yourself healthy — and it doesn't cost a cent

"Follow the water." This slogan guided the first NASA missions to Mars. Why? Because water is essential to survival.

Keep your body in smooth waters with H2O. Water in your body is a lot like oil in your car engine. It lubricates to keep things moving. It prevents waste from building up. And it stops the engine from overheating.

Without oil, your car would stop working. Without water, your body couldn't carry nutrients and oxygen to every cell in your body. And this is how it maintains your skin, hair, nails, body temperature, heart rate, and more.

You wouldn't let your car run out of oil, would you? But millions of people don't drink enough water each day, even though dehydration is one of the easiest conditions to avoid. Guzzling more water doesn't cost anything, and you'll see the benefits right away.

Dehydration hangs your health out to dry. Staying hydrated can help you avoid a long list of health hazards. That means you can spend less time with your doctor and lower your medical bills. Here's what you may miss by keeping a water bottle close.

- **Constipation.** When you drink water, where does it go? Straight through your digestive tract, of course. Your body soaks up the fluid in your intestines. But if you don't have enough water going through your pipes, hard stools that are difficult to pass get left behind.

- **Unbalanced blood pressure.** Once your intestines absorb water, they send it to your bloodstream to distribute to your thirsty organs. But if you don't have enough water, your blood volume goes down. That can lower pressure against artery walls, and a sudden drop in blood pressure can be dangerous. On the other hand, sometimes your body compensates by holding onto sodium, which can raise your blood pressure.

- **High cholesterol.** An internal drought may trigger a cholesterol hike. One study shows dehydration during fasting could cause a surge in bad LDL cholesterol. It's your body's way of protecting cell membranes from moisture and nutrient loss.

- **Poor stroke recovery.** High cholesterol and blood pressure both contribute to stroke risk. And since dehydration zaps water out of your arteries, your blood ends up even thicker. That raises chances of your condition worsening post-stroke.

- **Brain fog.** Experts aren't sure why dehydration affects your noggin. But your brain is about 75 percent water. So it makes sense that you need H2O balance for concentration, alertness, and short-term memory. Drink up to help your brain think better, remember more, and stay young longer.

- **Bad moods.** Dehydration isn't just linked to brain fatigue. Low fluid levels can really get you down. And according to studies, you only have to be mildly dehydrated to feel the effects. But feeling lethargic and down in the dumps is just the beginning. In one small study, dehydration in men actually increased anxiety.

- **Chronic pain.** Your body needs fluid to cushion and lubricate your joints to protect you from pain and wear and tear.

In fact, your cartilage contains water, which helps it stay firm and absorb shock. What's more, a recent study showed dehydration can increase pain sensitivity. That would make even a little discomfort feel a lot worse.

- **Kidney problems.** Your kidneys remove waste and extra fluid from your body, sending 'em straight to your bladder for removal. Water makes sure waste products, bacteria, and proteins move smoothly on the way out. Dehydration can lead to buildup and from there to dangerous infections, painful kidney stones, and in extreme cases, even kidney failure.

Pinch and press — 2 ways to test hydration

How do you know if it's time to break out the water bottle? If you have any of these signs of dehydration, start sipping.

- thirst and dry mouth
- muscle cramps
- headache and dizziness
- dark urine
- dry skin

Still not sure if you're dried up? Try one of these tests.

Skin pinch. Dehydration can curb your skin's ability to change shape and return to normal, known as skin elasticity. Gently pinch some skin on the back of your hand and stretch it up. When you release, the skin should bounce back into position.

Nail press. This test monitors blood flow to your tissues, which is a marker of hydration. Hold your hand above your heart. Apply pressure to your nail bed until it turns white, indicating that the blood has left the tissue. Remove pressure. If it takes longer than two seconds for the pink color to return, you may be dehydrated.

Trim your tummy with a simple switcheroo

Are you one sweet drink away from a shopping spree for bigger pants? Hang on to your britches, and make the switch to smarter sipping today.

Artificial sweeteners aren't such a sweet deal. Even though folks know sugar is bad for them, almost half of American adults drink at least one sugar-sweetened beverage every day. But what about low-calorie alternatives like aspartame, saccharin, sucralose, or stevia? They help keep your weight down, right?

Positive and negative studies have muddied the water. And the most recent review of seven randomized controlled trials — the gold standard in clinical research — showed inconsistent effects on weight loss.

But in the same review, researchers looked at 30 cohort studies — the kind used to establish links between risk factors and health outcomes, and reported bad news for sweetener fans. After analyzing 10 years of data from more than 400,000 participants, they found low-calorie sweeteners were linked to larger waists and hikes in blood pressure, diabetes, heart disease, and other health issues.

Experts suggest these fake sugars don't give you the sense of fullness your body expects, making you more apt to grab extra food throughout the day.

> How much water do you really need? It all hangs on your health, environment, and activity level. In general, experts recommend eight to 11 cups of fluids daily for women and 10 to 15 cups for men. Keep in mind, you get about four cups from other sources like food.

Swap out your go-to beverage for a flood of perks. So what can you do daily to watch dangerous abdominal fat melt away? Well, deadly belly fat is the first to go when you replace these sweet drinks with water.

"Regardless of how many servings of sugar-sweetened beverages you consume, replacing even just one serving can be of benefit," says Kiyah J. Duffey, co-author of a study that shows swapping sugary drinks for water can cut weight.

When you chug water, you nix the extra calories found in sweetened drinks. Maybe that's one reason drinking more water is linked to less weight gain.

Does your water glass need a little pizzaz? The simplest way to liven it up is to add a slice of lemon or lime. Go the extra mile, and infuse your drink with pineapple or strawberry chunks, slices of cucumber, or a few sprigs of mint. Or freeze fruit in ice trays to jazz up water with yummy kiwi or berry cubes.

Regular UTIs? End the cycle with 2 refreshing drinks

Oh no. Burning, back pain, discolored urine, and frequent trips to the bathroom with no relief. You have a urinary tract infection (UTI) — again. If only there was a way to cut down on repeat UTIs without pumping yourself full of antibiotics. You're in luck. Scientists say two refreshing beverages can get the job done.

Flush out bad bacteria with water. Here's a satisfying way to slash UTI risk in half. Add about six cups of water to your day, says a new study of women who are prone to the infections.

"While doctors have often recommended that women at risk for UTIs increase their fluid intake, it's never really undergone a prospective trial before," says Thomas M. Hooton, lead author of the study and clinical director of the Division of Infectious Diseases at the University of Miami School of Medicine. "It's good to know the recommendation is valid, and that drinking water is an easy and safe way to prevent an uncomfortable and annoying infection."

Guzzling more fluids raises the rate that bacteria gets flushed out of your bladder. Plus, it washes out any bacteria trying to sneak in from the vagina or rectum. This cuts down on opportunities for bacteria to attach to cells that line your urinary tract, which is how an infection gets started.

Cranberries clear up a sticky situation. Can cranberry juice really prevent UTIs? The research is mixed, but a recent study published by the *American Journal of Clinical Nutrition* offers hope.

Boston University researchers recruited 322 women who had experienced at least two UTIs in the past year. They drank either a cup of cranberry juice or a placebo drink every day for 24 weeks. The rate of UTIs went down by almost 40 percent in the cranberry group.

> Cranberries don't just prevent UTIs. The delightful juice also improves memory, blocks colds, and steadies blood sugar. You owe all this good stuff to polyphenols — plant compounds with antioxidant activity. Add two cups of cranberry juice to your day to jazz up your hydration routine and gain bonus benefits.

What does cranberry juice have that water doesn't? Well, not all bacteria is washed out by water. *E. coli*, the bugs that cause most UTIs, use finger-like projections to cling to the lining of your bladder. Here's how cranberries beat the bad guys.

- Proanthocyanidins. These flavonoids, found in plant foods, often act as antioxidants. They're the pigments behind that classic cranberry color. In this case, they actually keep bacteria from sticking to your bladder and creating an infection.

- D-mannose. This is a naturally occurring sugar your body does not absorb, but excretes in your urine. *E. coli* stick to it instead of the wall of your bladder. Then the pathogens get flushed out of your system before they can do any harm.

Scientists recently published results of the first randomized clinical trial examining d-mannose for preventing UTIs. Their findings look promising. Researchers included more than 300 women with recurrent UTIs. After six months, they found the d-mannose supplement was just as effective as nitrofurantoin, a standard antibiotic for preventing and treating UTIs.

Surprising workout trick helps you bag BP benefits

Don't drink more than six cups of water in an hour when exercising, says a training guide published by the U.S. Army. It makes sense. You don't want to waterlog your body before it has the chance to put all that fluid to work. But what about exercising? Should you spread it throughout the day, too?

Research says yes if you want to keep your blood pressure down.

Scientists asked folks with elevated blood pressure to walk briskly on a treadmill for three 10-minute sessions and one continuous 30-minute session. They kept track of their BP levels for 24 hours each time. And here's the shocker — they found the 10-minute sessions actually lowered blood pressure better.

Who knew walking 10 minutes at a time could get you healthier than half an hour of walking?

5 ways to stop a leaky bladder without surgery

Sometimes it happens when you run. Or when you cough. Or laugh. Other times, you just get overwhelmed with that got-to-go feeling — but it's already too late. Urinary incontinence, the loss of bladder control, strikes in many different situations. Good news — the solution might be easier than you think. Check out these natural ways to beat the leak.

If your bladder doesn't have the mastery it once boasted, your first instinct may be to drink less fluid. Don't. Experts say, to block a leaky bladder, you shouldn't skimp on the water.

That's because the less you drink, the more concentrated your urine will be. And undiluted urine can irritate your bladder and cause leakage.

What else can trigger an unwelcome escape? Here are four more irritants to look out for.

- Cut out caffeine. It's not just in coffee, either. You'll find it in soft drinks, teas, and chocolate.

- Avoid alcohol. Steer clear of the nightcap to control your bladder.

- Skip hot spices. Do your taste buds like the sizzle of peppers, curry, and more? Your bladder may not.

- Pass on acidic foods. Tomatoes, citrus, and even cranberry juice may be bad news.

'Egg-cellent' way to reuse cooking water

Pack more nutrients into soups and sauces by recycling water from boiled veggies, goes the old wisdom. But here's something really clever. Reuse cooking liquid from legumes as a vegan replacement for eggs.

Wait, that thick liquid you get from cooking dried beans? Yep. This stuff is called aquafaba.

Here's how you do it. Pour the aquafaba off the top of your cooked beans. It should be the same consistency as egg whites. Then start swapping.

3 tablespoons aquafaba = 1 whole egg

2 tablespoons aquafaba = 1 egg white

Muddied waters — the real meaning of your water bottle label

Pick up the nearest water bottle, and read the label. What exactly is 100-percent pure spring water? Or luxury artesian water?

Buying water in a bottle instead of getting it free from the tap can seem silly, even extravagant. But sometimes you do need to make that purchase. In that case, it helps to know what you're buying. Here are the most common label terms and what they legally stand for, according to the Food and Drug Administration (FDA).

Artesian. It's not synonymous with luxury. It just means the water was collected from a well that draws from an aquifer — an underground layer of rock and sand containing water. What makes it different from well water? When tapped, pressure causes the water level to rise above the top of the aquifer. That's it.

Spring. It's "100-percent pure" simply because 100 percent of it comes from an underground water source that flows naturally to the surface of the earth. The term doesn't say anything about quality.

Mineral. It has to have a certain amount of minerals and other organic material at its source, and minerals can't be added later.

Sparkling. This fizzy drink must contain the same amount of carbon dioxide it had when it emerged from the source. Unlike mineral water, the bubbly can be added back in after treatment.

Purified. The purification process removes chemicals and contaminants. Depending on the way the water was processed, the label may say "purified," "deionized," "distilled," or "reverse osmosis." Almost half of the bottled water sold in the U.S. is purified tap water, but the label only has to mention this if it doesn't meet the definition of one of the above terms.

To be kind to the environment and your wallet, go for tap water whenever possible. The Environmental Protection Agency (EPA) regulates safety. Plus, it's a few hundred times cheaper.

Watermelon

Bounce back post-workout with a refreshing melon

Watermelons are 92 percent water. No wonder early explorers used them as natural canteens. And while the water content makes them the perfect pre-workout snack for boosting hydration, this melon is also packed with nutrients that may help you even more after a tough exercise session.

Soothe exercise soreness with a tasty juice. Say you had a particularly hard-hitting workout. You felt great at first. But that was a day or two ago, and now your muscles are tender and stiff.

The discomfort you're feeling is called delayed-onset muscle soreness. And surprisingly, watermelon may put this pain in the past, says a small study published in the *Journal of Agricultural and Food Chemistry*.

One hour before exercise, a group of athletes drank either two cups of watermelon juice or two cups of a placebo drink. The next day, the lucky folks who got to sip watermelon juice were less sore.

Experts say the source of these perks is L-citrulline, an amino acid found in watermelon. It expands arteries, allowing more blood to flow throughout your body. So instead of standard shipping, your muscles get same-day speedy delivery of oxygen and essential nutrients. Maybe that's why studies also show L-citrulline supplements improve exercise performance.

Powerful antioxidant helps you recover faster. Antioxidants are fierce foes against cancer and heart disease. But did you know they can also protect against damage caused by exercise?

Take lycopene, an antioxidant famously found in cooked tomatoes. Experts used tomato juice in a study that showed lycopene can help your body recover from exercise.

Over two months, a small group of athletes subbed out fizzy sports drinks for the juice. It lowered markers of inflammation and muscle and tissue damage.

> Yellow watermelon, if you're lucky enough to come across one, contains four times more L-citrulline than red varieties. But which type is the king of lycopene? Red — it gets that bold color from the antioxidant, which doubles as a pigment. Both melons look similar on the outside, so check the label.

But here's more good news — especially if your taste buds prefer the sweet flavor of watermelon. Two slices have more lycopene than one cup of tomato juice.

To add juicy watermelon to your active lifestyle, slip them into smoothies ahead of an energetic exercise session.

Munch on watermelon for better blood flow

Someone once slung a watermelon at a Greek statesman during a speech. Legend has it, he placed it on his head and thanked the thrower for a helmet to wear as he fought the Macedonians. Here's a better way to make use of this melon. Chow down on it and boost your blood vessels.

Amp up artery action with a natural nutrient. Antioxidants in watermelon, like lycopene, help your ticker by protecting against damage caused by free radicals. But watermelon has another nutrient that also loves on your heart — the amino acid L-citrulline.

When your body gets L-citrulline, it converts it into another amino acid called L-arginine. This one can actually make nitric oxide, signaling arteries to relax, which boosts blood flow.

Magnificent melon cuts down blood pressure. It's a fact — more people die of heart attacks in the winter. That's because the stress of cold temps causes blood pressure to spike, making your heart work harder to pump blood. This often leads to less blood flow to the heart.

And so researchers designed a study to mimic cold weather conditions. Participants dipped one hand into 39-degree water while the experts took their blood pressure. BP went down for folks taking a daily watermelon extract containing 4 grams of L-citrulline and 2 grams of L-arginine.

"The pressure on the aorta and on the heart decreased after consuming watermelon extract," says Arturo Figueroa, lead author of the study published in the *American Journal of Hypertension*. "That means less overload to the heart, so the heart is going to work easily during a stressful situation such as cold exposure."

Get the Viagra effect with a dose of fruit. L-citrulline also boosts blood flow below the belt, which is important for men who want to get and maintain an erection.

To see how effective the amino acid is, researchers recruited a group of men with mild erectile dysfunction. The men first took a placebo for one month, then 1.5 grams of L-citrulline every day for another month. L-citrulline supplements improved erections and increased sexual activity.

Now to match the amount of L-citrulline used in the study, you would have to eat three and a half servings of watermelon a day. That's about 6 1/2 cups of diced watermelon. Unless you find a yellow watermelon, that is — one serving of that variety would do.

Supermarket secrets: pick a perfect melon every time

Lift your watermelon, and give it a good thump. Did it sound like a "pink," a "pank," or a "punk"? And what does that mean? Because the thump test isn't a foolproof method for choosing watermelons, you need a scientific way to decide which is best.

Watermelons that ripen fully on the vine make for the juiciest, tastiest snacks. When you're sorting through a pile of produce, you may avoid the ones that have ugly cream or yellow spots on the bottom. But that patch develops when the melon stays on the vine until it's ripe. So this is actually what you want to look for. White or light green patches mean the melon is underripe.

Plus, ripe watermelons please more than just your taste buds. As they ripen, they get redder. Redder melons mean more good-for-you lycopene.

Tasty tip-off — mouthwatering ways to use the entire melon

Visit a high-end department store in Japan, and you can buy a square watermelon — for a few hundred dollars. That's not the only downside to these strictly ornamental fruits. Because they are extremely underripe, you won't want to actually eat them. Regular watermelons, on the other hand, are entirely edible. You can savor every piece. Here's how to do it in style.

Try a new twist on the juicy middle. You've chopped it up and served it cold, but have you ever cooked a watermelon? Try it two new ways.

- Grilled. Slice a small melon into thick wedges, keeping the rind attached. Sprinkle on your favorite seasonings, such as salt, lime, and cumin. Grill two to three minutes on each side for a superb side dish.

- Dried. Remove the rind and slice your watermelon into 1/4- to 1/2-inch thick strips. Put these in a dehydrator for about eight hours. It could take longer — as much as 20 hours — but this watermelon jerky is worth the wait.

Crunch on nutritious seeds. No matter what you were told as a kid, the seeds won't grow into huge melons in your belly. But they will give you nutrients like magnesium, zinc, iron, and folate.

Many people like them roasted. With your oven set to 325 degrees, toast for about 15 minutes. Don't forget to add your favorite seasonings.

Tease your taste buds with yummy rinds. Watermelon rinds are good for more than just a decorative bowl. They're chock-full of L-citrulline. So try them pickled, juiced, or even stir-fried.

Wheat germ

Keep your noggin nimble with a scrumptious super germ

Are you as mentally sharp as you were just a few years ago? Test yourself with this teaser. Find three consecutive letters of the alphabet that can be added to ACK to form a six-letter word. Need a hint? How about this? Don't let age "hijack" your brain-power. Instead sprinkle a little wheat germ on your favorite foods to keep your mind sharp for decades to come.

Wise up to this wonder germ. Wheat germ — short for "ger-mination" — is the part of the wheat grain that sprouts into a new plant. Even though it's tiny, this seed is packed to the rafters with an important brain chemical called choline.

To work at peak performance, your brain needs a healthy amount of neurotransmitters that deliver messages from cell to cell. Choline is one of the elements your body uses to make the neurotransmit-ter acetylcholine. This chemical is vital for brain activities like attention, memory, learning, and muscle stimulation.

To put choline to the test, researchers evaluated almost 1,400 adults between the ages of 36 and 83. They found eating more choline-rich foods was linked to better verbal and visual memory.

Other studies agree — people with more choline in their bodies may process information faster, have stronger problem-solving skills, and be better at responding to new situations. And researchers speculate brain-boosting choline may turn out to be an effective tool in the fight against Alzheimer's disease.

Chow down on choline to get your fill of brain benefits.
Experts recommend 425 milligrams (mg) of choline per day for women and 550 mg for men. But a 14-year study showed American women only ate about 70 percent of the recommended amount. And men did even worse, taking in just 60 percent.

Your body produces some choline, but not enough for healthy brain function. You can pick up the slack with good nutrition, and that's where wheat germ comes in. Just one cup of toasted wheat germ provides a quick and easy 202 mg of the necessary nutrient. You can also score more by eating other choline-rich foods, such as beef liver, eggs, peanuts, and whole grains.

> A germ that grows good bones? A Norwegian study of almost 5,000 people discovered wheat germ's choline is a key nutrient for building better bone mineral density (BMD). The study showed that people with low choline levels were more likely to develop low BMD in their femoral neck — aka your hip — a common risk factor for hip fractures.

Reap 4 mighty nutrients from 1 tiny kernel

Sometimes it's good to be dense. Nutrient dense, that is. Wheat germ is one of those power-packed superfoods that provides you with a healthy serving of lots of nutrients, including the fantastic four listed below.

Manganese. This trace mineral is responsible for a laundry list of important functions, from making connective tissue and bone to supporting the hustle and bustle of your brain and nerves. It even helps monitor your blood sugar. And a 1-ounce serving of wheat germ — about four tablespoons — provides 186 percent of your daily value of manganese.

Thiamine. Its nickname is the "anti-stress" vitamin because it may strengthen your immune system and even improve your body's ability to handle stress. As one of eight B vitamins, thiamine's job is to maintain healthy skin, hair, and eyes. It also helps your nervous system run smoothly and keeps your brain function up to par. Sprinkle a tablespoon of wheat germ in your morning oatmeal to get close to 10 percent of the amount you need each day.

Sweet wheat reward: healthy germ from stem to stern

Wheat germ is not a whole grain. In fact, it's just a teeny nutritional nugget tucked inside the core of every grain of wheat.

The three parts of the kernel are the bran, endosperm, and germ. Bran is the outer layer of the kernel and contains a lot of the wheat's fiber. The endosperm holds most of the grain's starch. But the true prize? The germ.

That's where you'll discover a rich source of nutrients — vitamin E to protect cells from damage, choline for better brain health, phosphorous for strong bones and teeth, and zinc, a super disease fighter. And, as an extra bonus, wheat germ is a good source of protein.

Plus it's a breeze to work this nutritional gold mine into your menu. Add it to smoothies, use it instead of bread crumbs in your favorite recipes, or spoon it into yogurt for a crunchy treat.

Storage wars — keep it fresh in the fridge or freezer

To make sure your wheat germ stays fresh, keep it cool.

Wheat germ, both toasted and raw, is similar to vegetable, flaxseed, or sesame seed oil. If you leave it at room temperature for too long after it's been opened, it will spoil. So be sure you protect wheat germ's healthful nutrients like folate, vitamin E, and magnesium — just to name a few — by stashing it in the refrigerator after you open it.

Wheat germ will last about two weeks in the fridge. For even longer storage, tuck it away in your freezer for up to two months.

Magnesium. Your heart, muscles, teeth, bones, and kidneys all crave this mineral. Plus, magnesium manages your levels of crucial nutrients like copper, calcium, potassium, and vitamin D. An ounce of wheat germ gives you 17 percent of your daily value.

Selenium. This antioxidant wages war on free radicals that can harm your cells and cause problems like heart disease or cancer. Antioxidants like selenium can help wipe out free radicals and even undo some of the damage they cause. To get about a quarter of the selenium you need every day, add two tablespoons of wheat germ to your morning smoothie and sprinkle another one on your afternoon yogurt.

Wild salmon

Wild vs. farmed: the perfect pick for heart health

All salmon is the same — or so you would think. Take a quick
look around the fish section of your grocery store. You'll see fish
with labels like farm-raised, Atlantic, coho, and sockeye. They
all look pretty much alike, so why shouldn't you pick up the
cheapest one?

Farm-raised salmon is usually the least expensive, but it has
some serious downsides. It's more likely to be packed with pollutants that block the health benefits of omega-3 fatty acids.
Even worse, these harmful compounds actually raise your risk
of stroke.

Instead, you should seek out salmon who live their lives frolicking
in the open sea. Scan the labels and you'll find wild-caught fish are
lower in pollutants and packed with heart-healthy omega-3.

Fishy delight cuts stroke risk by 50 percent. Wild salmon
has two kinds of omega-3 fatty acids, docosahexaenoic acid
(DHA) and eicosapentaenoic acid (EPA). And experts say both
help you steer clear of strokes.

You suffer a stroke when blood vessels weaken and burst, or a
clot stops blood from getting to your brain. Both have devastating, even fatal, results. But if you're a fish lover, you may just
dodge the bullet. People who eat fish five times a week are half

as likely to suffer from strokes as infrequent fish eaters, several studies show.

High blood pressure can weaken your blood vessels, making dangerous clots and bursts more likely. But your friendly team of omega-3 fatty acids — DHA and EPA — work together to lower your pressure. Plus they reduce the stickiness of blood cells called platelets, so they're less likely to form clots.

Choose the right fat to manage your cholesterol. Waxy cholesterol is a big part of the sticky mess that clogs your arteries and leads to heart attack or stroke. Oddly enough, to help lower cholesterol, you need to eat more fatty foods. But forget the burgers and fries. Wild salmon and other fatty fish are the perfect choice because they have the right kind of fat — omega-3.

These fatty acids are the key to fish's heart-healthy powers. They work by increasing your good HDL cholesterol, particularly large HDL particles. Think of those particles as natural garbage men, seeking out harmful fats in your body and carrying them to your liver for disposal. The larger they are, the more fats they can remove, and the better they protect your arteries.

If you eat farmed salmon, trim off the skin and excess fat. That's where most toxins are stored. And try poaching, grilling, or baking your salmon on a rack to cook out even more fat.

A British study found that men who ate fatty fish for dinner every night for a month raised their HDL levels significantly compared to men who ate lean fish or meat. And in Finland, people who ate fatty fish three to four times a week had more large HDL particles in their blood than their friends who ate fish less often.

Fatty fish are fabulous in more ways than one. Heart health is not all wild salmon is good for. Omega-3 fatty acids have been proven to fight arthritis, Alzheimer's, and cataracts, too. A 3-ounce serving of this fishy delight boasts more than 2,000 milligrams of omega-3. Adding it to your dinner table is definitely a no-brainer.

Act FAST to get ahead of strokes

A stroke can sneak up on you without warning. And when one strikes, every second counts. So you need to know what to do immediately. To catch the early warning signs, remember the acronym FAST.

Face. Is one side of your mouth or face drooping?

Arms. Are your arms weak or hard to raise?

Speech. Are you slurring your words?

Time. As soon as you notice any of these signs, call 911 immediately.

If you can, take a full-strength aspirin while waiting for help. Studies show this drug can help limit the damage and reduce your risk for follow-up strokes.

Tame the flames of inflammation for OA and AD

Inflammation isn't all bad news. It's your body's way of fighting off infections, pollutants, and irritants. But if inflammation becomes a chronic problem, it can cause serious conditions like arthritis and Alzheimer's disease (AD). To head them off, you'll need to enlist one of nature's most powerful inflammation fighters — omega-3 fatty acids.

Strike back at arthritis with fishy delights. Wild salmon, sardines, mackerel, herring, bluefin tuna, halibut, sablefish, trout, and anchovies. That's a boatload of fish. And all nine are loaded with nutrients proven to get rid of joint pain and help increase your mobility.

A new study published in *Annals of the Rheumatic Diseases* found omega-3 fatty acids combat pain associated with knee osteoarthritis (OA). They work in part by blocking chemical messengers that trigger inflammation.

Scientists used to think you needed high-dose supplements to douse inflammation. But Australian researchers found that lower doses may be even more effective. In their study, people took a daily supplement that contained .45 grams of omega-3. That's a little more than what you'd get in a standard 1-gram fish oil capsule. Two years later, this group had less pain and better knee function than the group taking a dose 10 times higher.

Instead of popping a supplement, pop some fatty fish into your weekly menu. Just two servings will give your body more than enough omega-3 to help battle arthritis.

Dive into the sea to boost your brainpower. Salmon always find their way home. These fish are famous for migrating hundreds of miles back to the rivers where they were born. Scientists don't know why these fish have such amazing memories, but they think eating wild salmon can boost your brainpower, too. Plus help you fight Alzheimer's disease.

According to a University of Illinois study, eating a diet rich in omega-3 fatty acids helps older people at risk for AD improve their mental flexibility. Simply put, these nutrients help you switch between tasks more easily. And experts think this may be more important for day-to-day living than enhancing memory.

Scientists found that the omega-3 beefs up a part of your brain called the anterior cingulate cortex. Along with mental flexibility, this area is in charge of skills like goal-planning, problem-solving, and decision-making.

The study didn't give any guidelines on how much fish you should eat to get the full benefits. But just like for arthritis, twice a week is a good rule of thumb.

Limber up — this simple movement can help your joints

Adding inflammation fighters to your diet isn't always enough to stop arthritis pain. Sometimes you need a little extra push. And nothing works better than exercise. An easy workout can boost your mood, keep your joints flexible, and reduce your risk of falls.

Do you find you're a bit wobbly at times? Arthritis in your knees can affect your balance and make you more likely to take a tumble. This simple movement can help. Walk in a circle, gradually making it smaller and smaller. That will tighten the curve and make it more challenging to stay balanced. Do it every day for 15 minutes to help with fitness and stability.

Reel in some real protection against eye problems

Few movie moments are more magical than Dorothy's first glimpse of Oz. Who can forget the scene when black and white gives way to a colorful, beautiful world?

But if your eyesight is fading, every day can seem as bleak and drab as Dorothy's family farm. Wild salmon might be what you need to get your vision back on track — without taking a wild ride in a tornado.

See your way clear of cataracts. A clear web of proteins, called the lens, collects and focuses light on your retina so you can see. Over time light, ultraviolet radiation, and other irritants damage these proteins. Your body makes new ones, but the old, damaged cells don't leave your eyes. They build up in the center of the lens, eventually turning into cataracts that cloud your vision.

That's where wild salmon comes in. The omega-3 fatty acids in this fish are proven to protect your eyesight. One study found that people who eat at least a half gram of omega-3 fatty acids every day are 42 percent less likely to get cataracts. You can get four times that amount in one 3-ounce serving of salmon.

But this nutrient doesn't work alone — vitamin E plays a part as well. At least scientists think so. They know omega-3 raises the levels of HDL cholesterol in your blood. And HDL carries vitamin E molecules throughout your body, including to your eyes. They believe this powerful antioxidant helps fight off age-related damage known to cause cataracts.

Omega-3 will keep your peepers sharp. Think of your eye as the most advanced camera ever made — but it still needs film to work. Instead of traditional film, your eye-camera has light-sensitive tissue. At the center lies the macula, which helps your brain turn light into clear, sharp images.

As you get older, this tissue can be damaged by irritants or high blood pressure. Family history may play a part as well. If the macula breaks down, you'll experience wavy or blurred vision, a condition known as age-related macular degeneration (AMD).

In a certain form of AMD, abnormal blood vessels grow under your retina and distort your vision. No matter what type you have, you'll eventually lose your central vision.

But a healthy diet with plenty of omega-3 fats could be the key to saving your sight. According to one long-term study, women who got about 330 milligrams (mg) of omega-3 a day slashed their risk of AMD by 38 percent compared to those who averaged only 80 mg.

These nutrients protect your eyes by fighting off inflammation and helping to control your blood pressure. And experts think they actually stop rogue blood vessels from forming in your eyes.

The really good news? You don't even need to eat much fish to get the same amount of nutrients as people in the study. Half an ounce of salmon contains more than enough sight-saving omega-3 to fight AMD.

Vitamin B3 — a boon to your body

You shouldn't have to spend your golden years worrying about your health, fighting fatigue, and dealing with a fading memory. But if you eat right, you'll put yourself ahead of the game.

God has created a nutrient so powerful that it can crank up your energy, manage your cholesterol, fortify your mind, and more.

Era of the poodle skirt, the Bop — and niacin? If you had high cholesterol back in the 1950s, your doctor probably would have prescribed niacin, also known as vitamin B3. Turns out, it's one of the best natural remedies for high cholesterol, and doctors have been recommending it for years.

Niacin works by increasing your good HDL cholesterol, which helps whisk your bad LDL cholesterol out of your body. If you take it today, it's more likely to be a low dose to supplement a statin or other cholesterol-lowering drug. Scientists have found that high doses can cause dangerous side effects like bleeding, infections, or even death.

Feeling a little flushed? This mild side effect can occur with just 30 milligrams (mg) a day. The bottom line — don't take a niacin supplement without talking to your doctor first.

Fortunately, niacin from food is much safer. You'd have to eat 65 pounds of salmon to get a dangerous dose. That's quite a bit, even for salmon fanatics. Experts recommend getting about 15 mg of niacin every day. You'll be more than halfway toward your goal by eating a delicious 3-ounce salmon fillet for dinner.

Take advantage of a natural energizer. Niacin plays a big role in keeping you energized. Like the other B vitamins, it helps your body change carbohydrates into sugar for fuel.

Think of niacin like a car's engine. The food you eat is the gas that makes the car (your body) run. But you need something to help convert that gas into mechanical power. Niacin sets off the chemical reactions that transform food into the energy that keeps you going.

B3 — a powerful brain booster. Do you find yourself feeling confused and forgetful? Shortages of niacin can do that to you. Even more scary — it causes long-term damage like dementia, too.

Adding salmon to your menu can help. A niacin-rich diet has been linked to a lower risk of Alzheimer's disease. According to a study of close to 4,000 Chicago residents, people who got the most niacin from foods were least likely to develop Alzheimer's. They also stayed mentally sharp longer than those with low niacin intakes.

The credit goes to this B vitamin's brain-building powers. Niacin plays an important role in your brain, helping with processes like DNA repair, nerve cell growth, and cell communication.

Omega-3 and niacin: how do they stack up?		
Type of salmon	Omega-3 fatty acid content (per 3-ounce serving)	Niacin content (per 3-ounce serving)
king (Chinook)	1,822 mg[*]	8.5 mg
pink	1,237 mg	7.2 mg
sockeye (red)	1,210 mg	5.7 mg
coho	947 mg	6.8 mg
keta (chum)	807 mg	7.2 mg

*milligrams (mg)

Fresh, frozen, or canned? Smart answers to a fishy dilemma

Don't fall for the myth that fresh fish is always better. Other healthy options are hiding in your grocery store if you know where to look.

Frozen fish — a nutritional powerhouse and more. Unless you caught the salmon yourself, it's been previously frozen. All wild-caught fish is frozen on commercial fishing boats. That means anything you see in the seafood section that looks "fresh" has been thawed out, so it will only last a day or two in your refrigerator.

But don't worry about quality. Modern freezing technology works fast to help lock in flavor and freshness. An added bonus — it helps kill parasites and food-borne bacteria. Just remember to thaw frozen fish properly. Leaving it overnight in the refrigerator is the best way to make sure your fish is flavorful and fabulous.

Canned salmon — a healthy (and cheap) alternative. If you want to enjoy salmon without spending big bucks, head over to the canned food aisle. A small can of salmon costs less than $2. And it's almost always wild-caught, but read the label to be sure.

This cheap pantry staple is an excellent source of nutrients, too. A 3.5-ounce can of pink salmon has almost 1,500 milligrams (mg) of omega-3 fatty acids. Use a large can of salmon in your recipe, and you'll get a whopping 8,000 mg of healthy omega-3.

And unlike fresh or frozen salmon, canned salmon is high in calcium. A small can of salmon packs almost as much calcium as a glass of skim milk. The secret is all the tiny bones mixed in. They're soft enough to eat, so don't be afraid to mash them into your favorite salmon croquettes or casseroles.

Don't get duped into buying farm-raised fish

Wild salmon costs a pretty penny, but some stores and restaurants don't want to pay a premium to sell the good stuff. So guess what? They substitute the cheaper farmed salmon for wild and charge you big bucks for lower-quality fish.

Four out of 10 salmon sales may be deceptive, according to a recent study. To make sure you're getting the real deal, follow these simple tips.

- Look for products that list specific types of salmon instead of generic labels. Products that give the name, like Chinook or coho, are less likely to be mislabeled.

- Don't buy fresh salmon out of season. The fishing season runs from May to September, so salmon sold during the winter is probably farm-raised.

- Bargains are usually busts. If the price seems too cheap, chances are it's not actually wild salmon.

- Because of overfishing, the only salmon that comes from the Atlantic is farmed.

Yogurt

This one-two punch knocks out osteoporosis

What do yogurt and super glue have in common? Believe it or not, they were both discovered by accident. The first yogurts popped up thousands of years ago, when folks attempted to store milk in warm climates. To their surprise, the fermented food actually tasted great. These days, scientists realize yogurt has benefits beyond tickling your taste buds. And one of the things it's best for is warding off brittle bones.

Don't skimp on this mineral if you want a strong skeleton. Your bones and teeth play host to about 99 percent of the calcium in your body. That's how they stay so strong under pressure. But what happens if you don't get enough?

To balance mineral levels in a calcium recession, your body takes it from bones. And if a temporary recession turns into a long-term depression, your bones can become brittle — a condition known as osteoporosis. Unfortunately, sometimes the only warning you get is a broken bone.

So keep up calcium levels with yogurt. A single cup of low-fat yogurt contains almost half of your daily recommended dose of the mighty mineral.

Load up on prebiotics — you're eating for more than one. When you eat, you're not just feeding yourself. You're also feeding trillions of bacteria that live in your gut. Don't worry, most of these germs are actually your friends — they help you digest food, use nutrients, and even fight off diseases. This community, known as your microbiome, may hold the key to staving off brittle bones.

If your gut bacteria aren't healthy and happy, your body might not absorb nutrients properly, calcium included. You can help by feeding them prebiotics. Your body can't digest these fibers, but they are a special treat for the bacteria in your microbiome. Two types of prebiotics in particular will help make sure you're absorbing all the calcium you need.

- **Inulin.** This fiber found in chicory root is often added to yogurt to make it thick and creamy, but it has the added benefit of making your yogurt healthier, too. A yearlong study found that adding 8 grams of inulin to your daily diet increased calcium absorption by almost 20 percent in a small group of young people. Look for mention of inulin, chicory root, oligofructose, or fructo-oligosaccharides (FOS) on the label.

- **Galacto-oligosaccharides (GOS).** These prebiotics have been shown to increase calcium absorption in post-menopausal women. They are actually created from the lactose in milk, and Japan and some countries in Europe already have fermented dairy products — like yogurt — that contain GOS. Adding galacto-oligosaccharides to dairy products is seen as a promising way to improve health. Although they're not available everywhere, it's something to look for in the future.

In the meantime, to help increase calcium absorption from yogurt and other dairy products, make sure you eat plenty of foods rich in GOS prebiotics. You'll find these compounds in lentils, chickpeas, kidney beans, lima beans, and green peas.

Got milk? Dairy can help you duck diabetes

Your diet is your first line of defense against type 2 diabetes. But if you only focus on avoiding sugary snacks and fatty fare, you'll overlook some powerful foods. Researchers think yogurt and other dairy products could help you get the upper hand on this common condition.

Pick the right protein source to slash your risk of diabetes. Does it really matter where your protein comes from? Well, recent studies show that people who eat too much meat are more likely to get type 2 diabetes. On the other hand, folks who get more protein from yogurt and other dairy products are less likely to develop the disease.

Is protein the main menace? Maybe not. The iron in red meat may be partially to blame. High blood levels of this heavy metal actually increase your body's production of free radicals. These feisty atoms can harm your pancreas and keep it from making enough insulin. And all the salt and nitrates added to processed meat may also put your pancreas in the danger zone.

But dairy products contain a triple threat to diabetes risk — milk proteins, vitamin D, and calcium — all of which are thought to be protective.

Go "pro" to keep your blood sugar under control. Many yogurts contain friendly bacteria called probiotics. They help you

Don't make the mistake of buying just any yogurt. A lot of brands pasteurize their products at high temperatures, which kills the good bacteria. Read the label to find yogurt with the "Live and Active Cultures" seal. That means it meets the probiotic standards set by the National Yogurt Association. And for the best benefits, eat it before the expiration date.

ward off diabetes by getting to the gut of the issue — skyrocketing sugar levels.

In a recent study published in the *American Journal of Clinical Nutrition,* researchers asked overweight women to eat either regular yogurt or a yogurt with active probiotic cultures. After 12 weeks of adding the creamy treats to their main meals, those who ate the probiotic yogurt had better insulin sensitivity. That means their bodies didn't have to work as hard to balance blood sugar.

Researchers boosted the probiotic yogurt with *lactobacilli* and *bifidobacteria* strains. When you visit the grocery store, look for these strains plus a label showing it has live and active cultures.

Go face-to-face with yogurt's skin-smoothing benefits

Loaded with calcium and "good" bacteria, yogurt helps your insides run smoothly. But the power of this tangy treat doesn't end there.

Fed up with spending big bucks on overpriced night creams? Look no further than your fridge. Fermented dairy products can boost skin health, say studies. And it doesn't matter if you eat them from a bowl or dab them on in front of the mirror.

Simply squeeze half a lemon into a cup of plain yogurt and stir. Smooth the mixture over your face before going to bed, avoiding your eyes. Then refrigerate the leftovers for future use. You should notice healthier-looking skin in a few weeks.

'Legen-dairy' treat supports your ticker and tummy

Imagine your local store sold pills that promised to help you lower cholesterol and melt away fat. You'd probably think it was too good to be true. But it turns out, they sell something pretty close — yogurt. Researchers are discovering this tasty treat may be exactly what you need to keep a healthy heart and a slim waist.

Your stomach — the key to combatting high cholesterol. The way to your heart is through your belly — literally. Choosing the right foods is one of the best ways to battle rising cholesterol. And few foods are better fighters than yogurt containing beneficial bacteria, shows a recent study published in the *American Journal of Clinical Nutrition*.

Overweight women ate 14 ounces of either low-fat yogurt enriched with active probiotic cultures or conventional low-fat yogurt every day for 12 weeks. At the end of the study, those who snacked on the probiotic kind had significantly lower cholesterol.

The powers of probiotics come from their ability to bind to cholesterol and sweep it out of your body. That keeps your gut from absorbing the cholesterol into your bloodstream where it can build up in your arteries.

For the study, researchers enriched the probiotic yogurt with at least 10 million colony forming units (CFUs) of *lactobacillus* and *bifidobacteria*. Look for these added strains as well as the words "Live and Active Cultures" on your supermarket yogurt.

Dig in daily to tip the 3 in your favor. Yogurt can do more than protect your heart, it can also pull a disappearing act on the extra pounds. Studies show people who eat more yogurt tend to be skinnier than those who don't.

The secret to yogurt's fat-trimming potential might be calcium. Past research shows this mineral actually keeps your body from building up fat while helping you burn it off at the same time.

Plus experts say overweight people often don't have the right balance of gut bacteria, leading to slow digestion and weight gain. Good thing probiotic yogurt is packed with good bacteria — the perfect snack to get your microbiome on the right track.

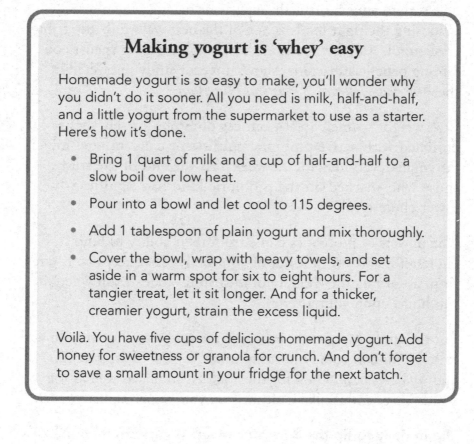

Making yogurt is 'whey' easy

Homemade yogurt is so easy to make, you'll wonder why you didn't do it sooner. All you need is milk, half-and-half, and a little yogurt from the supermarket to use as a starter. Here's how it's done.

- Bring 1 quart of milk and a cup of half-and-half to a slow boil over low heat.

- Pour into a bowl and let cool to 115 degrees.

- Add 1 tablespoon of plain yogurt and mix thoroughly.

- Cover the bowl, wrap with heavy towels, and set aside in a warm spot for six to eight hours. For a tangier treat, let it sit longer. And for a thicker, creamier yogurt, strain the excess liquid.

Voilà. You have five cups of delicious homemade yogurt. Add honey for sweetness or granola for crunch. And don't forget to save a small amount in your fridge for the next batch.

Beat the blues with a white delight

Move over double chocolate ice cream. There's a new comfort food in town, and it's actually good for you.

Long thought of as a way to build better bones and keep trim, yogurt's benefits may extend to your mood. Who would have thought a simple trip to the dairy aisle could pep up your step?

High-fat yogurt keeps you in high spirits. A recent study from Spain says eating whole-fat yogurt may help ward off depression. Women who ate a half cup of the yogurt at least seven times a week were less likely to develop depression than those who ate the same amount less than once a week. Low-fat yogurt didn't have the same effect.

Scientists don't know what causes depression, but they do say it may be linked to low-grade inflammation and a lack of folate in the diet. That's where whole-fat yogurt steps in. It contains more folate than the fat-free variety. And experts think healthy fats fight inflammation.

More fat doesn't mean more calories. High-fat yogurt won't pack on the pounds. In fact, an 8-ounce container of plain, whole-milk yogurt contains just 149 calories. Oddly enough, the same amount of low-fat yogurt has 154 calories. Pull out your reading glasses, scan the nutrition label, and you'll find the reason why. The low-fat version has almost 6 more grams of sugar than the high-fat kind.

Bacteria boost your brain. Fermentation, which gives yogurt that classic tangy flavor, is caused by friendly bacteria. These good guys may also put you in a good mood. That's because certain strains of *lactobacillus* help keep your brain in balance, studies say.

For more information on how good bacteria might ax anxiety and depression, see *Don't let your gut feelings get you down*, in the *Lactobacillus* chapter.

Swap out sour cream with Greek yogurt

About to make your favorite dip and realize you're out of sour cream? Or maybe you're looking for a healthy, lighter alternative. The good news is you can use Greek yogurt in just about any recipe that calls for sour cream.

For a change of pace, top off a slightly cooled baked potato with a thick, creamy dollop of Greek yogurt. Then add fresh chives, parsley, and black pepper.

Whole-milk Greek yogurt works best in baked products. Use an equal amount in place of sour cream in biscuits, breads, and cakes. You'll get a less dense, slightly tangier treat.

But don't mix yogurt directly into simmering sauces, stews, or soups. Its lower fat content makes it more likely to curdle than heavy creams. Wait until you're ready to serve before you add it to your dish.